MW01627020

A Clinical Atlas of Endodontic Surgery

Ralph Bellizzi, DDS, FICD, FACD
Colonel, Dental Corps
Consultant in Endodontics to the Surgeon General of the United States Army
Director of Endodontics,
One Year Advanced Educational Program in General Dentistry,
Ft Benning, Georgia
Former Director,
Endodontic Residency Training, Madigan Army Medical Center,
Tacoma, Washington
Diplomate, American Board of Endodontics

Robert Loushine, DDS, FICD
Lieutenant Colonel, Dental Corps
Assistant Director of Endodontics,
One Year Advanced Educational Program in General Dentistry,
Director of Dental Education, USA Dental Activity,
Ft Benning, Georgia
Diplomate, American Board of Endodontics

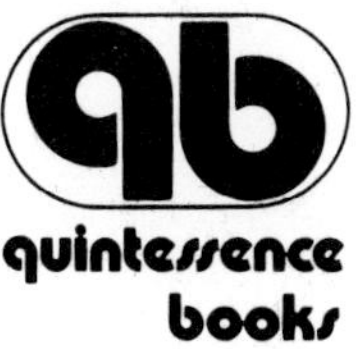

Quintessence Publishing Co, Inc
Chicago, London, Berlin, São Paulo, Tokyo, and Hong Kong

The opinions and assertions herein are the private views of the authors and are not to be construed as official or as reflecting the views of the Department of the Army or the Department of Defense.

Library of Congress Cataloging-in-Publication Data

Bellizzi, Ralph,
A clinical atlas for endodontic surgery/Ralph Bellizzi, Robert Loushine.
p. cm.
Includes index.
ISBN 0-86715-234-6
1. Endodontics. 2. Endodontics—Atlases. I. Loushine, Robert.
[DNLM: 1. Root Canal Therapy—methods—atlases. WU 17 B444o]
RK351.B45 1991
617.6'342'00222—dc20
DNLM/DLC 90-9245
for Library of Congress CIP

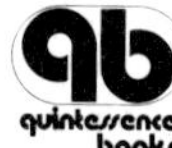

© 1991 by Quintessence Publishing Co, Inc, 870 Oak Creek Drive, Lombard, Illinois 60148-6405
All rights reserved.

This book or any part thereof must not be reproduced by any means or in any form without the written permission of the publisher.

Books Editor: Laura G. Peppers
Production Manager: Kim Vander Steen
Production Editor: Kristen Trotter

Composition: Graphic World, St Louis, MO
Lithography, printing, and binding: Toppan Printing Co (S) Pte, Ltd, Singapore
Printed in Singapore

Dedication

Docendo discimus
"We learn by teaching"

To my wife, Monique, and daughters, Jacqueline and Claudine, for the countless hours lost to them in a pursuit of truth and professional excellence.

Ralph Bellizzi

To my wife, Sandy, and our children, Amy and Bethany, for their love and support during the time this book was prepared.

Robert Loushine

Contents

Foreword

by L.K. Bakland

Surgery for endodontic problems has been performed for centuries. Historical references to trephinations and replantation of teeth indicate an early recognition that surgical approaches for the relief of pain and swelling from diseased teeth could be beneficial. In recent years, the advancement of endodontic techniques has included a better understanding of the role surgical procedures play in achieving successful results.

The topic of endodontic surgery, while generally recognized as an important modality within the specialty practice, has not been extensively covered in the form of textbooks, and opportunities for advanced training in surgical techniques have been very limited. This atlas of endodontic surgery by Drs Ralph Bellizzi and Robert Loushine will provide an excellent opportunity for endodontists and other dentists with an interest in these procedures to obtain an almost hands-on experience in basic surgical techniques in endodontics.

The book is clearly intended as a clinical atlas to demonstrate both basic and advanced surgical endodontic procedures. As such, that text employs a clear, concise style with an innovative approach. It is assumed that readers have become familiar with endodontic surgery on at least a basic level via endodontic textbooks and other sources. Therefore, this atlas may serve as a most useful adjunct to other texts.

There are several aspects of this text that readers will find very helpful. The illustrations are arranged so that they clearly demonstrate procedures and concepts. For instance, in the five chapters dealing with specific surgical areas, each step in the procedures is delineated using both graphic and photographic illustrations. To supplement the illustrations, concise guidelines are included that emphasize both what to do and what to avoid.

Other areas that many will appreciate are extensive descriptions with illustrations, and information on sources — of armamentaria, flap design, suturing, and relief of pressure from abscesses and cysts. An area not always included in texts or chapters on endodontic surgery, namely postsurgical complications, is covered in adequate detail to be a significant source of reference particularly to clinicians with minimal experience. Each potential complication is described with recommendation for management.

This atlas is a refreshingly innovative contribution to the endodontic literature. It does not purport to be an all-encompassing text, but instead is a clear and concise guide to basic endodontic surgical procedures. In that it succeeds admirably, and Drs Bellizzi and Loushine are to be congratulated on their fine work.

Leif K. Bakland, DDS
Associate Dean and Professor of Endodontics
Loma Linda University

Foreword

by G.R. Hartwell

Doctors Ralph Bellizzi and Robert Loushine are to be commended for their outstanding preparation of this clinical atlas of endodontic surgical procedures. Each chapter begins with a "straightforward" explanation of the important considerations that must be foremost in the operator's mind before performing the procedures illustrated in a step-by-step manner in the chapter. There is also a very logical sequence to the way the procedures are presented to the reader. The photographs are outstanding, and each illustrates the point for which it was intended ("One picture is worth a thousand words"). This is definitely a "how-to" text that will prove useful to the novice as well as the experienced clinician.

In today's clinical practice of endodontics, surgical procedures play an extremely important role in the management of endodontic problems. Endodontists and general dentists alike are confronted on a daily basis with cases that, for a variety of reasons, are not amenable to nonsurgical endodontic treatment. If these teeth are to be retained, surgical endodontic procedures must be performed. This atlas will prove to be a most helpful guide to anyone who chooses to perform these procedures. The chapters on molar surgery are outstanding and contain many helpful hints and illustrations for even the most experienced surgeon. The information presented makes this atlas a "must" for every endodontic surgeon's library.

Gary R. Hartwell, DDS, MS, FICD, FACD
Professor of Endodontics
Medical College of Virginia

Preface

The degree of difficulty and the complexity of the endodontic cases we are currently challenged to treat demand all our resources to include surgical endodontics. This atlas is an outgrowth of this challenge. Lengthy periods of time were spent not only on what this atlas would be, but also on what it would not be.

We conceived a text that would appeal to those students, teachers, and clinicians who perform basic endodontic surgical procedures, as well as those who deal with more complex and demanding cases. Our purpose was not to create a text burdened by a clutter of illustrations or lengthy discussions, but rather to design a simplified format that provides positive reinforcement through a written text coupled with descriptive photographs.

We initiated this atlas on the assumption that the clinician has demonstrated the ability to master basic surgical skills and comprehend those didactic subjects that are part of the curriculum both at the graduate and undergraduate levels. We encourage the reader to supplement the atlas with those basic science texts when required.

In this atlas we departed from tradition and designed a text that takes us away from standard formats in order to emphasize basic principles frequently lost in the verbiage of more detailed texts. Our approach was to create an atlas that presents itself as a pictorial "road map" of surgical techniques commonly used in endodontics.

Each chapter is used as a building block for subsequent chapters. Basic surgical techniques are developed from routine and simple cases to more complex cases. Chapters begin with a brief narrative outlining our objectives. This narrative is developed around a section of surgical technique notes that comprise helpful hints and observations presented in a sequential order for each case. We also introduce a format that uses brief and concise phrases (called "bullet statements") that are found either under or between the illustrations pertinent to each statement.

The illustrated cases were selected to represent basic concepts in an actual clinical setting while reflecting our philosophies and techniques. In its entirety, the atlas is designed to be a quick reference and review, ideally suited for the office or classroom. The value of this atlas lies in the step-by-step photographic layout along with clinical salient features that allow you to assimilate and retain the necessary knowledge to perform the various surgical procedures.

We have been very fortunate as co-authors to have in common a deep commitment to both teaching and sharing with others. We sincerely hope our readers will benefit as much from reading this text as we have gained from writing it.

Acknowledgments

We have found, as have many authors before us, that the preparation of a book owes its final form to those who molded and shaped our earliest professional experiences. We would like to express a debt of gratitude to our mentors and facilitators: Elmer J. Neaverth, John W. Harrison, Gary R. Hartwell, Roger N. Weller, and James C. Kulild.

During the tenure of our clinical, didactic, and professional experiences many of our colleagues have contributed their ideas and constructive criticism. For those who told it like it was, we are indebted to Frederick Cox, James Deemer, Elias Drobotij, Paul Dargon, Sylvester Robinson, William Corbin, Arvid Olson, Michael MacPherson, Kurt Obeck, and Gerald McMahon.

Without the exceptional surgical support of our tireless and overburdened staff, this pictorial atlas could not have come to fruition. We are indebted to Darlene Gottfried, Sigrid Osman, Kathryn Murphy, and Jewell Styles.

The preparation of any text is a tedious and time-consuming task. To those special individuals who have helped us through the maze of confusion, rewrites, and corrections, we would like to recognize Margarette Brown and Karen Heid for their advice, encouragement, support, and administrative expertise.

The superb artwork for graphics and illustrations must be attributed to Charles Pagan, Ron Bell, and Kevin Fifield.

Logistic support during preparation could not have been accomplished without the seasoned experience of James Gulsby and Herbert Johnson.

1 Presurgical Preparation

It is at this time, before therapy, that lines of communication are established between clinician and patient. A rapport is developed that allows both patient and clinician to mutually share concerns before surgery.

The patient is informed why he or she has been referred, the nature of the problem, and the techniques that will be used to deal with each situation. One of the most important parts of the presurgical conference is a frank discussion of the prognosis and postsurgical sequelae that may or may not accompany surgery. Anatomic structures that may be encountered are discussed. Written instructions, both preoperative and postoperative, are used as adjuncts to complement the narrative, which might otherwise inadvertently be forgotten by the patient during the course of the discussion.

Presurgical technique notes

Referral data

Ensure that all referral data are on hand. Review with the patient what he or she has been told about the case; elicit his or her expectations and establish the chief complaint. Compare this information with your referral data. Frequently, very valuable diagnostic data can be gained that was previously overlooked.

Record review

Review for accuracy and update all vital statistics, to include name, address, date of birth, primary health care contact point, telephone numbers, (both at home and work), as well as social security number, insurance provider, and next of kin or guardians.

Medical history review

Before you start any therapy, review the patient's present and past medical history. The existing history must be reviewed, signed, and updated. Conduct a general survey of the major body systems: cardiovascular, respiratory, gastrointestinal, urogenital, endocrine, and central nervous. Pay particular attention to such areas as:

1. Past and present medications
2. Allergies
3. Bleeding tendencies
4. Past and recent hospitalizations
5. Infectious diseases (eg, tuberculosis, hepatitis, herpes, human immunodeficiency virus)
6. Rheumatic fever
7. Diabetes
8. Cardiovascular review
   - Hypertension (take a base line reading and record it before therapy)
   - History of recent or past myocardial infarction
   - By-pass surgery
   - Valve replacement
9. Cancer
10. Immune suppressive therapy
11. Epilepsy
12. Glaucoma
13. Asthma

Any other health-impaired conditions suspected should be ruled out by a physician before therapy.

Preoperative radiographs

Periapical radiographs (straight-on views and altered angulation, either from the mesial or distal) should be reviewed before any surgical procedure is attempted. A panoramic radiograph is recommended for posterior surgery.

If a referral radiograph is sent, it should be kept and made part of the permanent record. However, a new radiograph is always taken by the clinician before any form of therapy.

Altered angulations reveal additional canals and/or roots, which may or may not have been obturated; fractures; position of pins and posts; and to some degree the density of any previous obturation.

The panoramic radiograph is important, especially in posterior surgery, because it reveals anatomic landmarks such as the inferior border of the mandible, mental foramen, mandibular canal, size and extent of any pathology, and the anterior, posterior, and inferior extension of the maxillary sinuses.

An occlusal film is suggested for palatal root procedures. Altered vertical angulations are taken when required to indicate facial and lingual positions of the mandibular canal.

Diagnosis

The diagnosis is confirmed based on clinical data available, radiographs, past and present dental history, signs and symptoms, and diagnostic testing. A preliminary periodontal examination with a periodontal probe is performed and any significant problems are recorded. The patient is informed, the examination is documented, and a copy is sent to the referring dentist to complete the record.

Case presentation

After the data have been collected, reviewed, and assimilated, a diagnosis is confirmed. The patient is informed and the following are discussed:

1. Rationale for surgical intervention
2. Type of surgical technique
3. Flap design
4. Bone removal
5. Root exposure and therapy (vertical root fracture may be present)
6. Flap replacement and suturing
7. Followup
8. Prognosis (not a 100% guarantee)

This conference is usually brief and to the point but covers the essential items that patients are concerned with and that are consistent with current trends in risk management. Remember, allow the patient to ask any questions concerning the course of treatment.

Postrecovery sequence

Instruct the patient on the possibility of several postsurgical complications that might result:

1. Swelling
2. Pain
3. Paresthesias
   - Mental nerve
   - Mandibular nerve
   - Lower lip
4. Maxillary sinus involvement
5. Bleeding
   - Hematoma formation
   - Facial discoloration

Informed consent

When considering a surgical procedure, the clinician must allow the patient to participate in the decision-making process regarding his or her treatment. Informed consent has evolved out of numerous interpretations by the courts and state legislatures.

These repeated interpretations have made it difficult for us to formulate a simple, uniform doctrine of informed consent that fulfills all the legal requirements. State statutes vary regarding informed consent, and clinicians should consult their state statutes before drafting their own particular informed consent forms (*American Association of Endodontists Communique,* Vol III, July 1986, p 4).

Preoperative patient preparation

Use of barrier techniques by the clinician and staff (ie, gloves, masks, eye protection, surgical gowns, and caps) as well as patient draping are discussed with the patient. Because the patient is conscious during these procedures, this discussion and description of sterilization techniques reduces anxiety and patient apprehension. At the same time, this discussion enhances patient confidence and the realization that the patient is benefiting from the state of the art of current standards for infection control.

Prior to surgery, premedication for medical conditions and anxiety may be prescribed as required. Chlorhexidine antiplaque mouthrinse *(Peridex)* has been found to be very effective in reducing plaque formation. It is used as a presurgical rinse beginning 1 day before surgery and as a postsurgical rinse until suture removal. Analgesics are prescribed before surgery as a convenience to the patient. The medication can be taken 1 hour before the procedure, thereby taking advantage of preoperative dosing, delaying the onset of postoperative pain (prophylactic analgesic effect). Narcotic analgesics should be prescribed when required; however, the nonsteroidal anti-inflammatory drugs (NSAIDs) have proven extremely effective and should be considered initially by every clinician in an effort to distance ourselves from prescribing addicting medications.

Surgical preparation

The patient is instructed on the importance of good oral hygiene. He or she is told to floss and brush the teeth the night before surgery. The use of an antiplaque rinse after brushing is emphasized. On the morning of surgery, the patient is instructed to eat a normal breakfast, brush and floss the teeth, and rinse with an antiplaque mouthwash.

Elective procedures are scheduled early in the morning and at the beginning of the week.

Before the patient is draped, anesthesia is administered and the appropriate level of anesthesia is obtained.

The clinician and assistant are gowned, capped, and gloved. The patient is draped and capped and protective eye wear is placed. Lip lubricant is applied to include the corners of the mouth; this prevents drying and cracking. Lubricant is reapplied during the surgical procedure as required.

2 Armamentarium

The armamentarium used for endodontic surgery is built around basic instruments used for the majority of routine oral surgical procedures. Each surgical tray is a reflection of clinical experience, individual philosophies, and new ideas that direct the clinician's approach to therapy.

Many new adjuncts used in endodontic surgery involve current technologies that expand the use of existing instruments. In turn, these instruments enhance the clinician's ability to expand and amplify surgical techniques, thus providing the patient with treatment options not previously available.

It is axiomatic that the degree of difficulty in the cases we currently treat has increased. Re-treatment and surgical intervention are considered important aspects of therapy. Surgical procedures are apt to become more difficult the further posteriorly the surgical site is located because we encounter anatomical structures that may or may not be limiting. Such space limitation tests our ability to locate and prepare root apices, place retrograde restorations, and suture soft tissue back to its original position. The most salient aspects of endodontic surgery, especially in the posterior region, are access, visibility, and the use of current technologies that allow us to effectively perform the type of surgery described in this atlas.

Surgical technique notes

Basic surgical tray setup

The setup should reflect simplicity and minimize clutter. It should be organized before surgery in the order and sequence that each instrument will be used during the surgical procedure. Special instruments that the clinician feels reflect his or her particular needs should be placed in the correct sequence.

Fiberoptic light source

The limited confines of the oral cavity reduce the effectiveness of the overhead light source and compromise visibility. This is especially true the further posteriorly the surgical site is located. A fiberoptic system attached to a retractor provides a point source of light on the surgical field. As a result, the light source remains constant and free from tissue impingement.

High-torque surgical drill

This instrument uses torque rather than speed. Torque is the rotational equivalent of force in a linear motion. It represents how much force a rotating shaft, such as a bur, can exert on another object. This system removes thick bone with ease and does not burnish it. It does not clog or scatter debris under the flap. It has a digital control that facilitates operational expediency without vibration or intense noise common to other systems that rely on compressed air. This electric motor–driven system also prevents the phenomenon of cervicofacial subcutaneous air emphysema. This phenomenon can occur when typical dental handpieces are used that have air turbines that exhaust their air into the surgical field. This forced air is capable of dissecting its way through the fascial planes.

Miniblade and scalpel

This system represents a departure from the conventional blade size and handle used in oral surgery. The advantages of this system are the small handle and blade size, which facilitate interproximal and intrasulcular incisions in confined and irregularly shaped areas. The pencil grip of the handle allows ease of manipulation as well as sensitive and precise control during incision.

Periosteal elevator

Traditionally, the pointed, spear-shaped end of the periosteal surgical elevator is used. This is placed interproximally, usually crushing interproximal bone during reflection. An effective alternative is the use of a no. 4 Molt curet. Its sharp cutting edge facilitates periosteal reflection and its convex surface enhances atraumatic tissue reflection. It is used to initiate reflection in the midportion of the vertical incision. The broad end of the standard periosteal elevator can be used in a similar manner. However, it is broader and thicker and does not have the same sharp edge for elevating periosteum as effectively as does the no. 4 Molt curet.

Retroapical file holder

Orthograde instrumentation often is not possible because of main canal blockage where the apical portion of the canal appears patent; in this instance a retroapical file holder can be used. An endodontic file size is selected; it is seated and firmly secured in the locking end of the apical file holder. The length is measured and the instrument file handle is disengaged from the instrument shaft. It can now be used in a filing motion apically until the desired depth and canal size are achieved. This technique is not a substitute for conventional orthograde instrumentation techniques.

Microhead handpiece

The comparison size to a conventional handpiece head is obvious. The small head size facilitates manipulation and placement at the surgical site. The microburs provide an advantage when dealing with small and narrow cross-sectional diameters of resected roots. The microhead handpiece is easily adapted to conventional handpieces and can be sterilized with ease.

Hemorrhage control

The surgical site can be isolated prior to retrograde obturation by using *Nu Gauze,* bone wax, *Gelfoam,* or *Surgicel,* which act as physical barriers and are easily adapted to the pathologic defect. After isolation, the apical preparation is dried using a cut paper point held by cotton pliers. The hemorrhage control barrier is removed before final closure and suturing.

Retrograde amalgam setup

A separate retrograde amalgam setup allows all instruments to be consolidated into one pack. It facilitates sterilization and is available on demand. The mini-amalgam carrier enhances the placement of retrograde amalgam in restricted surgical sites. The size and quantity of the amalgam used can be varied.

Conventional amalgam carriers are too large and expel large amounts of excess amalgam; this contributes to apical splatter in the surgical site. Custom-prepared amalgam condensers are an asset to apical condensation because they are small and can be adapted to suit most apical preparations. They are prepared from standard no. 23 sickle explorers. The tips are cut at 2-mm intervals as per choice or case selection. The cut ends are flattened using a sandpaper disk to remove any flash or spurs that may be present. This provides a clean flat surface for condensing the amalgam.

Retrograde *IRM* setup

IRM (Intermediate Restorative Material) as an alternate retrograde filling material is gaining in popularity. Its ease in mixing and placement is considered a decisive advantage. The apical preparation is not altered from that of the Class I or slot preparation used in retrograde amalgam preparations. The retrograde setup consists of a sterilized glass mixing slab, spatula, plastic instrument, and condenser of choice.

Visual magnification

Use of a fiberoptic point light source and improved access resulting from the use of a high-torque handpiece have allowed a new dimension of visualization that has not been previously explored. Current systems of visual magnification also provide an unparalleled view of the surgical site, with emphasis on visualizing the root apices. There are many systems to choose from. Prices vary depending on the quality and precision of the optics, the addition of custom prescription, and special operational features such as flip-up capability, telescopic angulation, and different working ranges. Each system should be explored and a choice made to reflect the clinician's particular needs.

Oral hygiene

Plaque control and healthy gingival tissues are a prime requirement whenever surgical procedures are performed. In addition to proper brushing and flossing, the use of chlorhexidine rinse is recommended before and after surgery. *Peridex* is an oral rinse containing 0.12% chlorhexidine gluconate that has been shown to be effective in inhibiting supragingival plaque growth. It is a microbicidal that reduces both aerobic and anaerobic organisms. *Peridex* has been used within the field of periodontics for short-term duration (1 to 2 weeks) following periodontal surgical procedures when the patient has difficulty in maintaining optimum oral hygiene because of postsurgical discomfort.

As a presurgical rinse, *Peridex* has proven to facilitate plaque reduction and enhance gingival health. Used as a rinse the evening before surgery, the morning of surgery, and 1 hour before surgery, it is the closest we can come to a "presurgical scrub." After surgery the patient is advised to rinse three times a day for 3 to 5 days as part of home care oral hygiene.

Postsurgical discomfort at a recently created surgical site can frequently deter patients from tooth brushing and maintaining oral hygiene. The use of a soft disposable toothbrush *(Toothette)* already impregnated with a mint-tasting dentifrice and activated by saliva is a valuable adjunct for maintaining oral hygiene. The *Toothette* gently removes surface plaque and debris from the surgical site; the patient's regular toothbrush can be used in the remainder of the oral cavity. Patients are prescribed enough disposable *Toothettes* for a 3- to 5-day period.

The *Toothette,* when used in conjunction with *Peridex* mouthrinse, proves to be an unbeatable combination for improved oral hygiene; it is an option previously not available to patients.

Basic Surgical Tray Setup

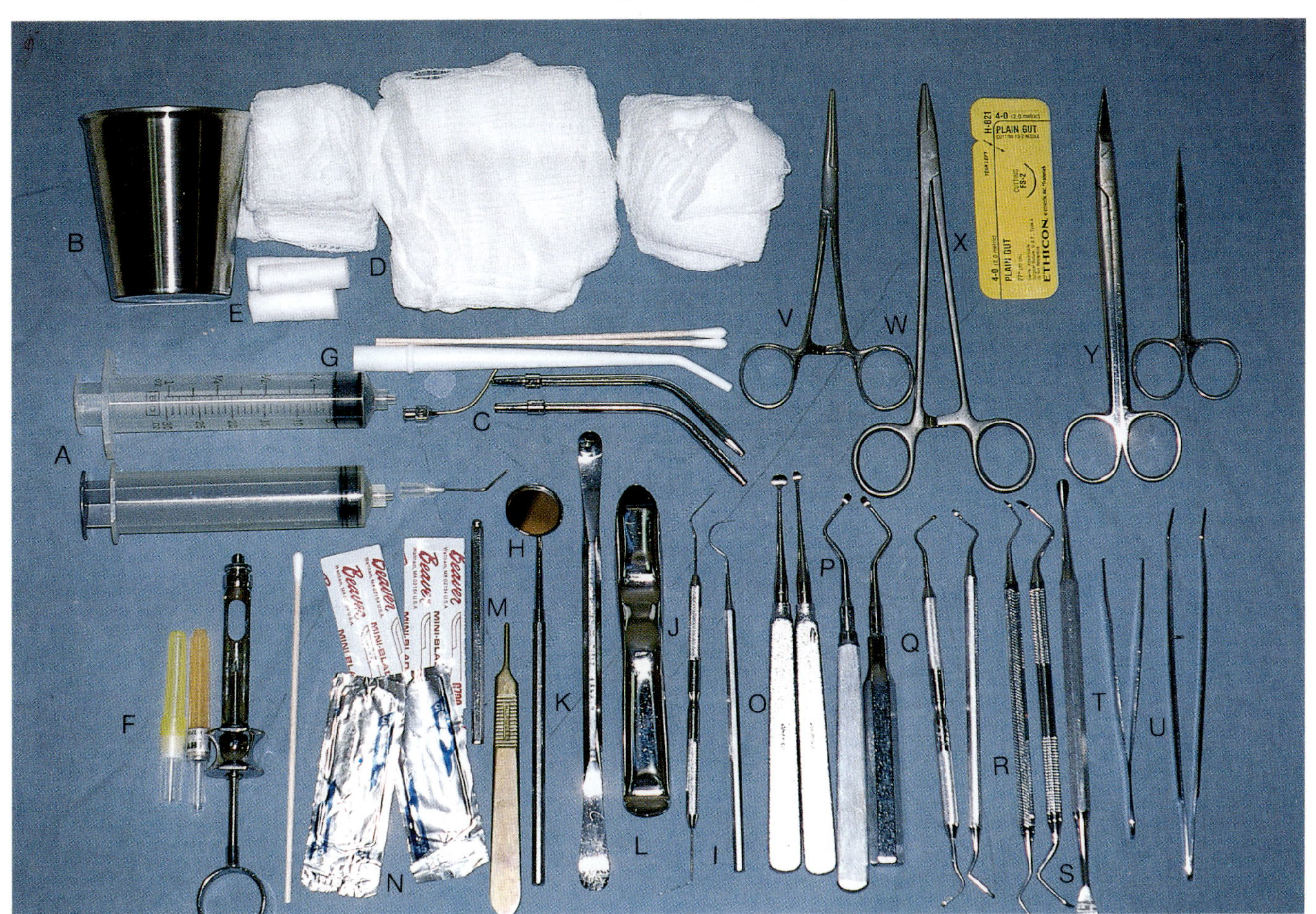

A, Irrigating syringes (2); **B,** Irrigation receptacle; **C,** Suction tips (2); **D,** 2 × 2 gauze/4 × 4 gauze; **E,** Cotton rolls/cotton pellets; **F,** Anesthetic syringe and needles; **G,** Cotton-tip applicators; **H,** Mirror; **I,** No. 23 explorer; **J,** Endodontic explorer; **K,** No. 23 Seldin retractor; **L,** Minnesota retractor; **M,** Surgical blade handle (2); **N,** Surgical blades (no. 15); **O,** Molt curets (no. 4, no. 2); **P,** Curets (5L, 5R); **Q,** Excavators (33L, University of Oregon 4); **R,** Periodontal curets; **S,** Bone file; **T,** Tissue forcep; **U,** Cotton pliers; **V,** Hemostat (curved); **W,** Needle holder (7-in. Hegar-Mayo); **X,** Suture material (4-0 silk/4-0 gut); **Y,** Scissors (iris, dean).

Supplemental items not shown: carpules of anesthetic and irrigation solution (sterile saline), surgical drill, surgical-length burs, biopsy bottle, fiberoptic attachment for the no. 23 Seldin retractor.

Fiberoptic Light Source

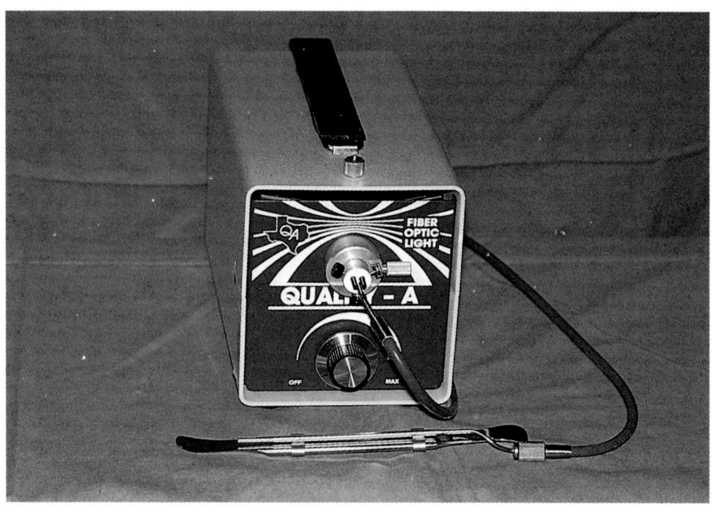

- Power console.
- Fiberoptic cord with wand attachment.
- Retractor.

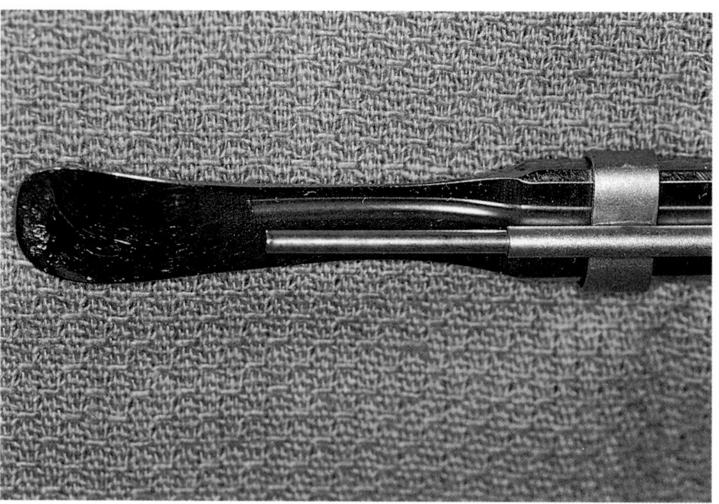

- Adapter clip on no. 23 Seldin retractor.
- Adjustable wand in position.
- Directs unimpeded light to surgical site.

Surgical Drill

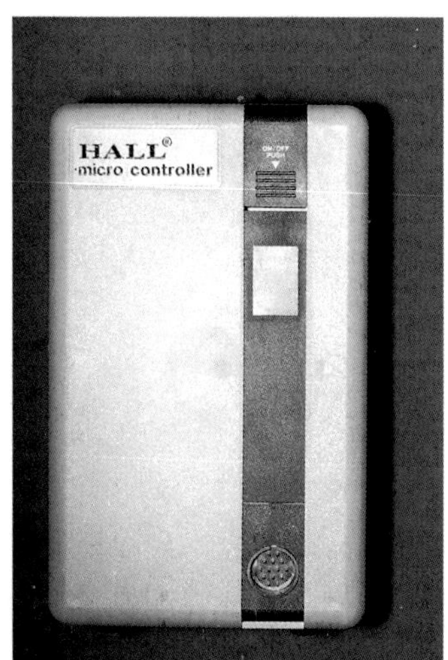

- Power console.
- Electric motor drive.
- Compact and portable.
- Absence of compressor and air hose reduces noise level.

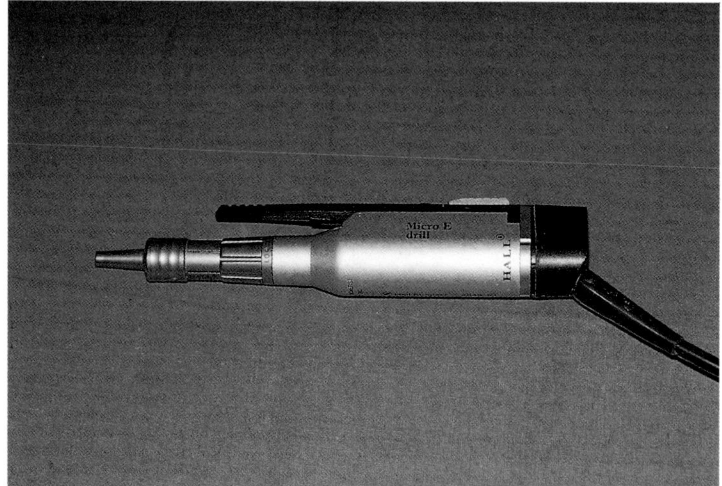

- High-torque delivery system.
- Torque facilitates unimpeded bone removal.
- Finger-tip control.
- Removable bur guard.
- Steam sterilizable.

Miniblade Scalpel System

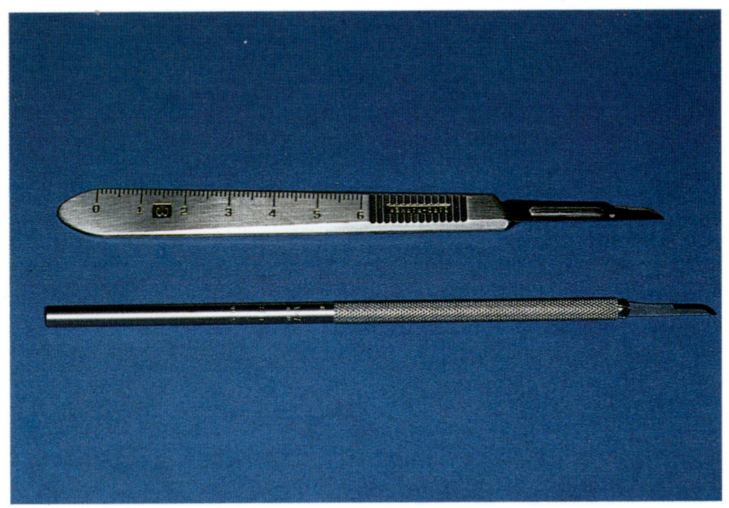

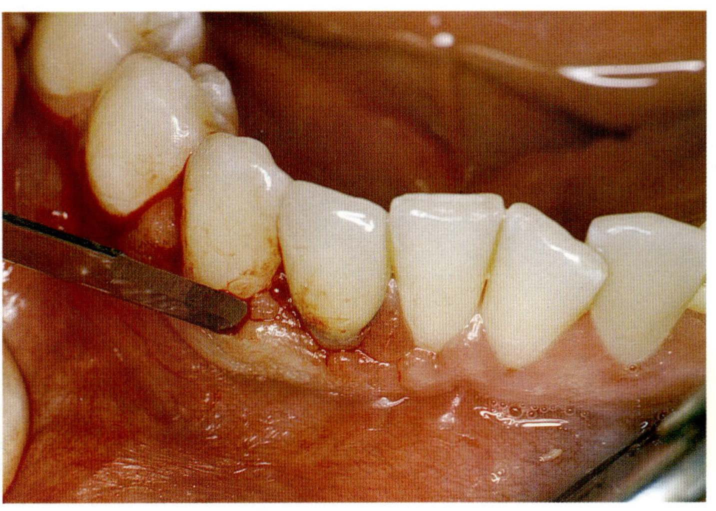

- Standard no. 15 blade and *Bard Parker* blade handle compared with the miniblade and handle.

- Miniblade facilitates intrasulcular and interproximal incisions and enhances control in irregular areas.

Periosteal Elevators

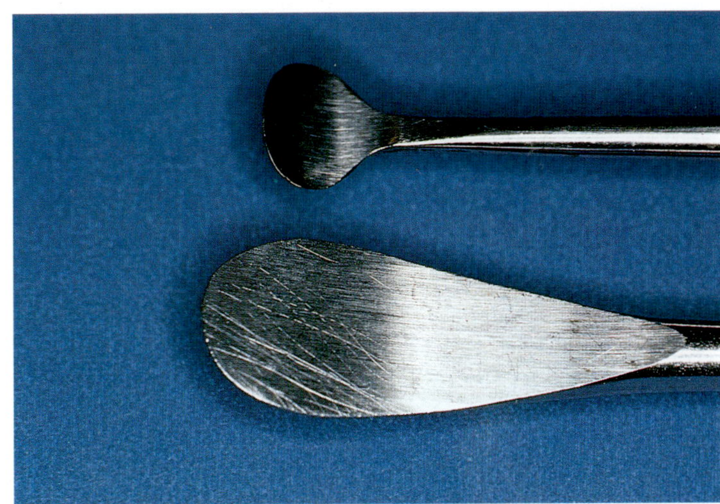

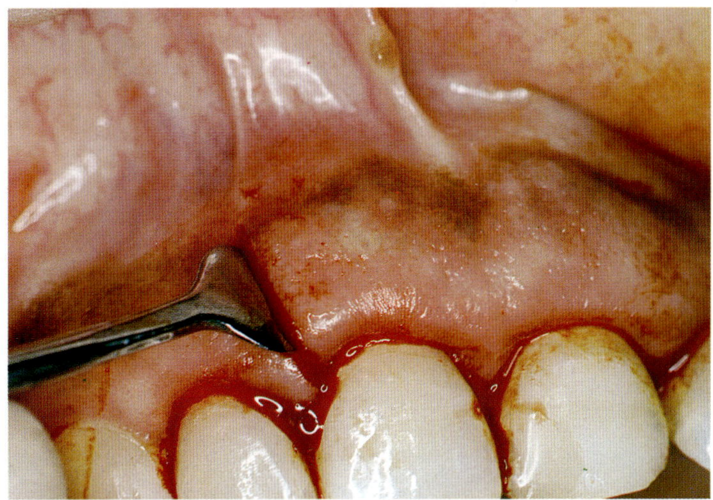

- The no. 9 periosteal elevator compared to the no. 4 Molt curet.

- No. 4 Molt curet:
  - Used as a periosteal elevator
  - Has sharp cutting edge
  - Cutting surface facilitates tissue reflection
  - Small size enhances interproximal tissue reflection without impinging on the interproximal bone

Reflection

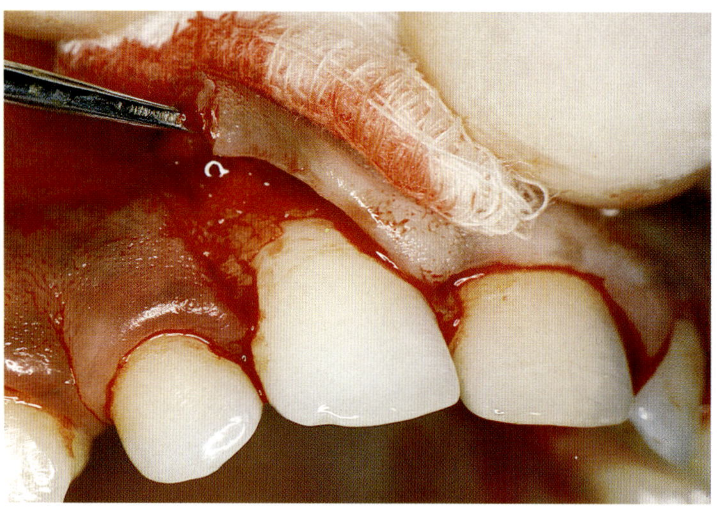

- No. 4 Molt curet.
- Quartered gauze backing:
  - facilitates tissue reflection
  - prevents flap perforation

Retroapical File Holder

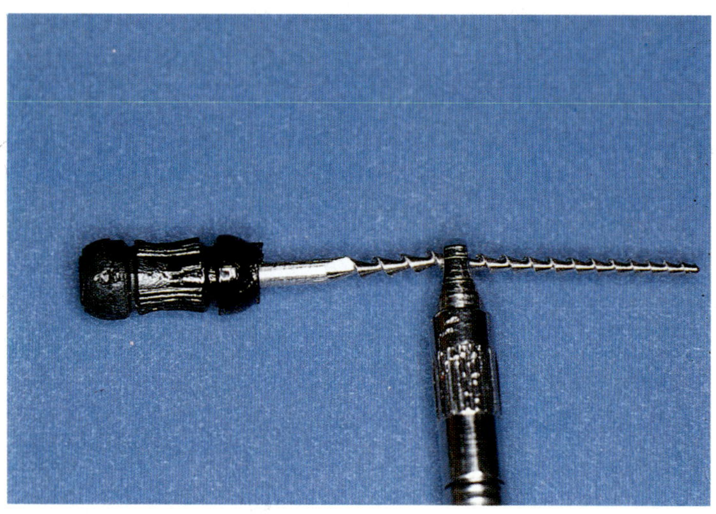

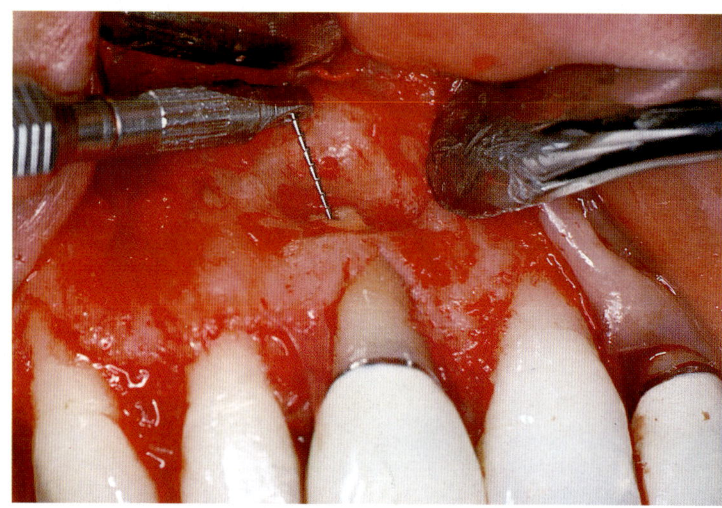

- Primary usages:
  - post and cores with incomplete apical obturation
  - canal blockage that prevents conventional coronal cleansing and shaping
- Not a substitute for orthograde instrumentation.

Microhead Handpiece

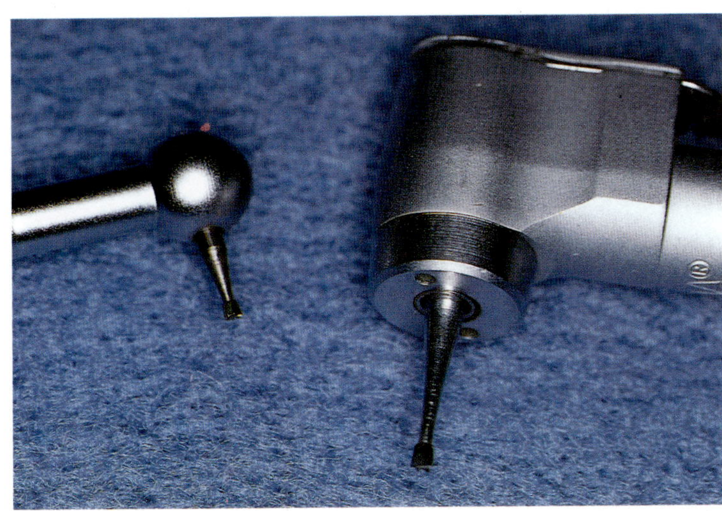

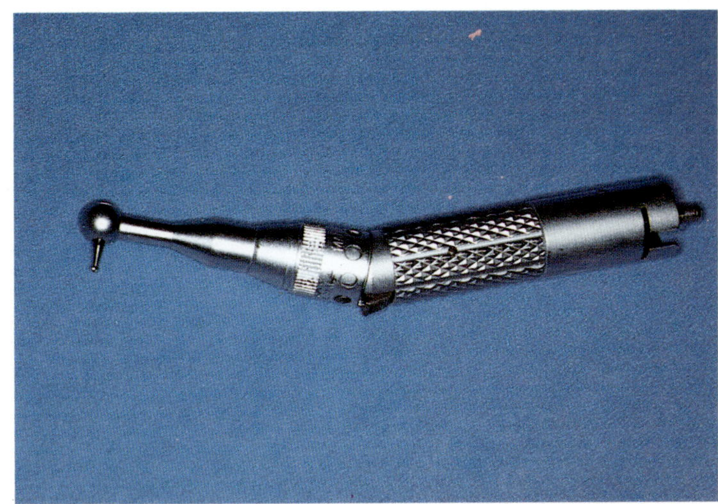

- Microhead and microbur facilitate root end preparation in confined areas.

Retrograde Amalgam Setup

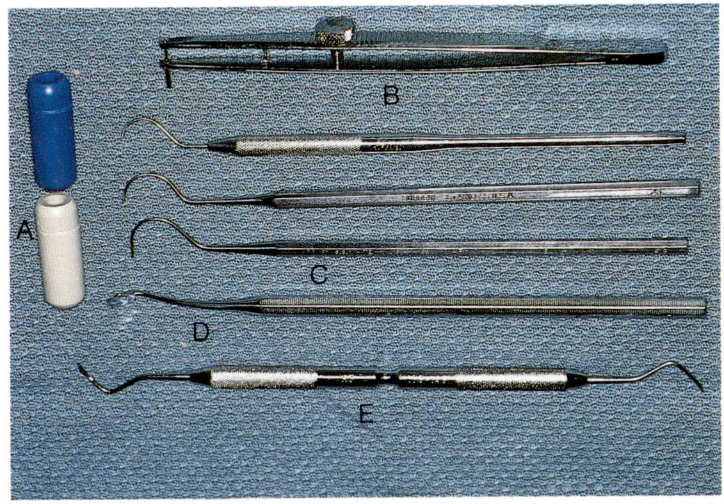

- **A,** Amalgam capsules.
- **B,** Miniamalgam carrier.
- **C,** Modified amalgam condensers.
- **D,** Apical retrograde mirror.
- **E,** Amalgam carving instrument.

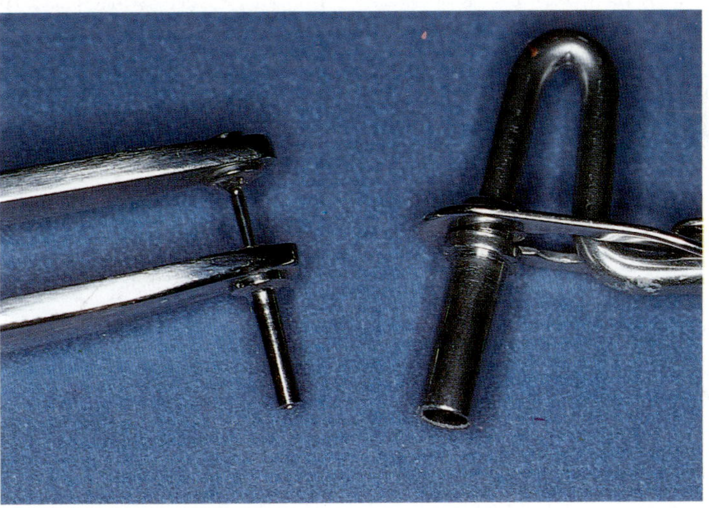

- Minicarrier compared to small end of a standard amalgam carrier.

Placement of Retrograde Amalgam

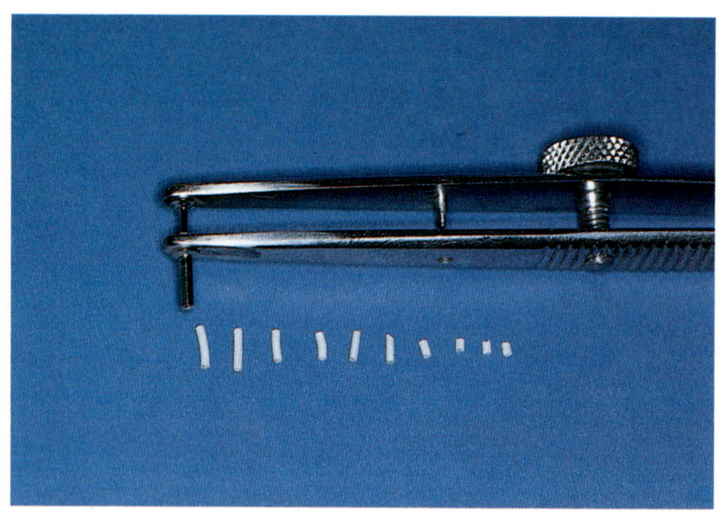

• Adjustment knob controls amalgam increment size.

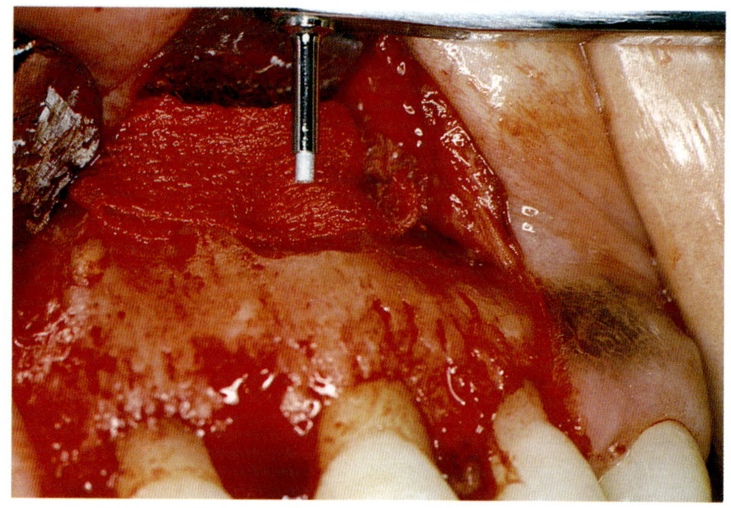

• Miniature size facilitates amalgam placement into retrograde preparation.

Retrograde Amalgam Condensers

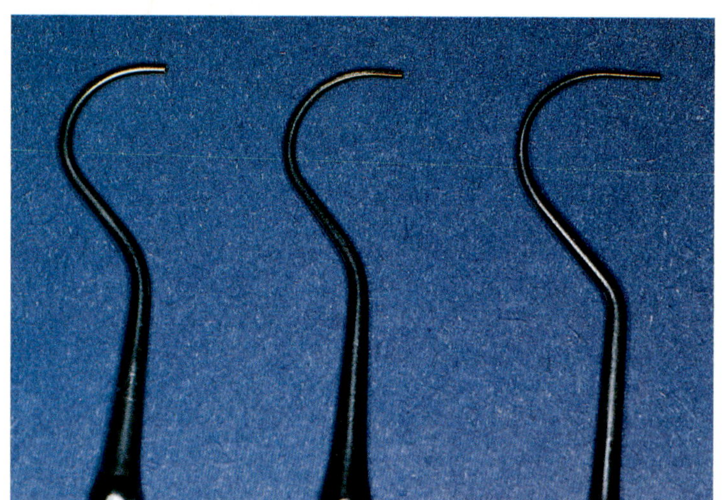

• Modified from standard no. 23 explorers.

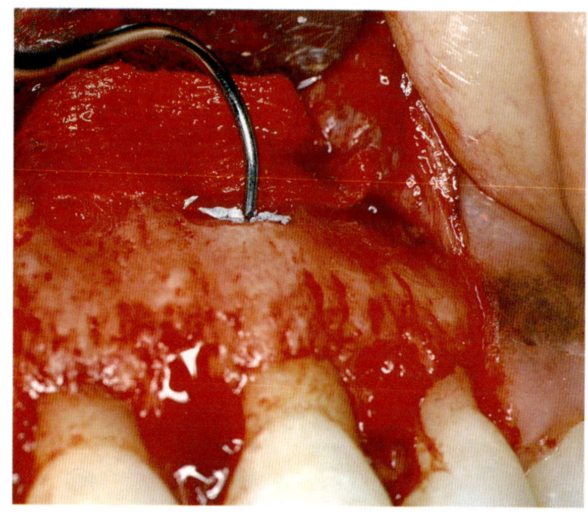

• Tips cut at 2-mm increments and ends flattened.
• Variable sizes suitable for case selection.

Retrograde IRM Setup

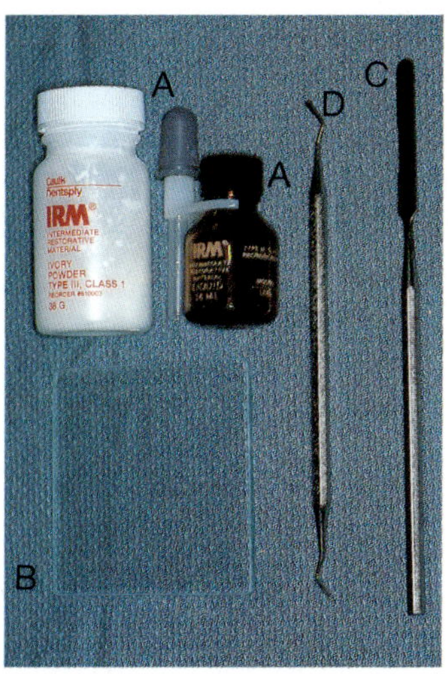

- **A**, *IRM* (powder, liquid).
- **B**, Glass slab.
- **C**, Mixing spatula.
- **D**, Plastic instrument (1-2).

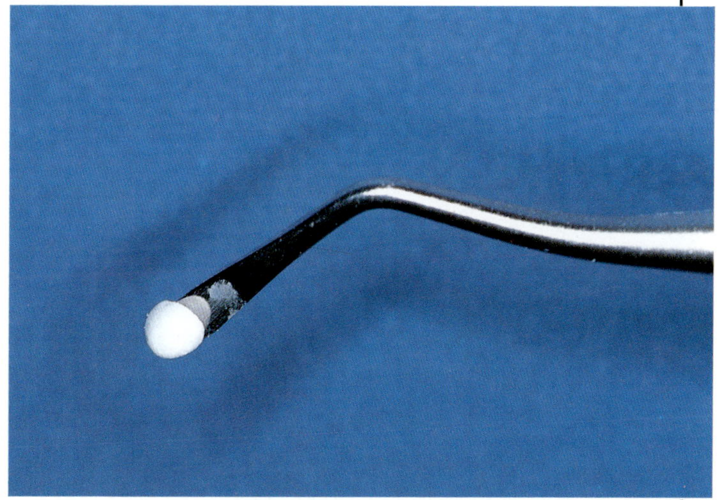

- Mixed *IRM* ready for placement.
- Material is easy to handle and place.

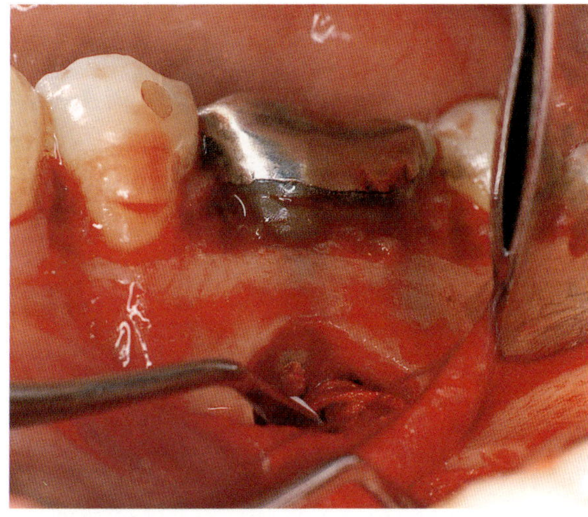

- Prepared surgical site and apical preparation receiving *IRM* for the retrograde obturation.

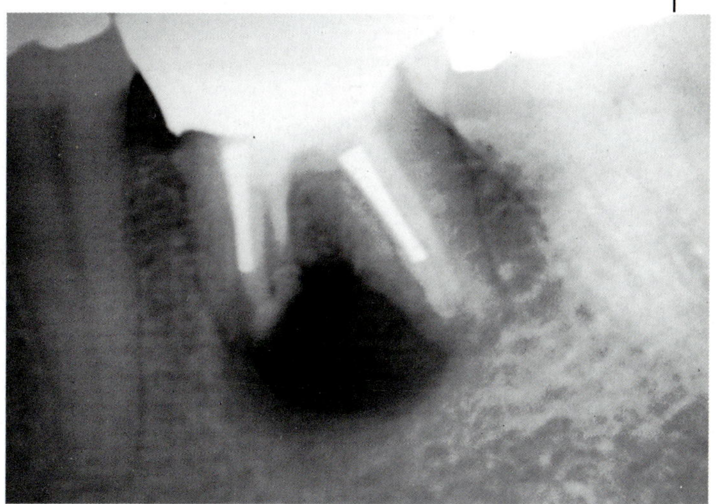

- Radiograph shows *IRM* in situ.

Retreatment Using an *IRM* Retrograde Obturation

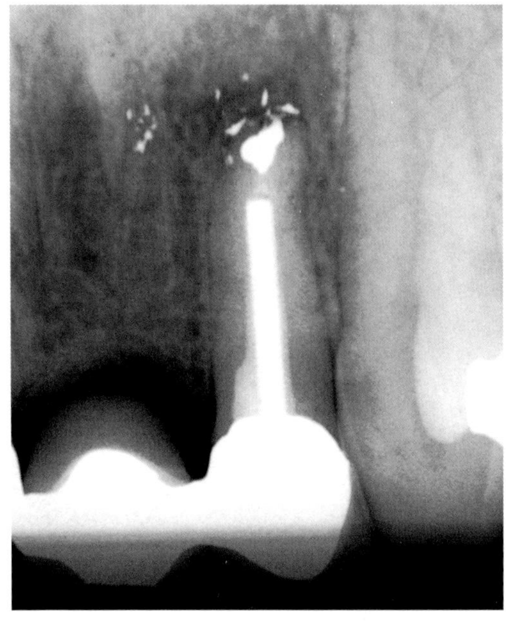

- Failed retrograde amalgam of 2-year duration.

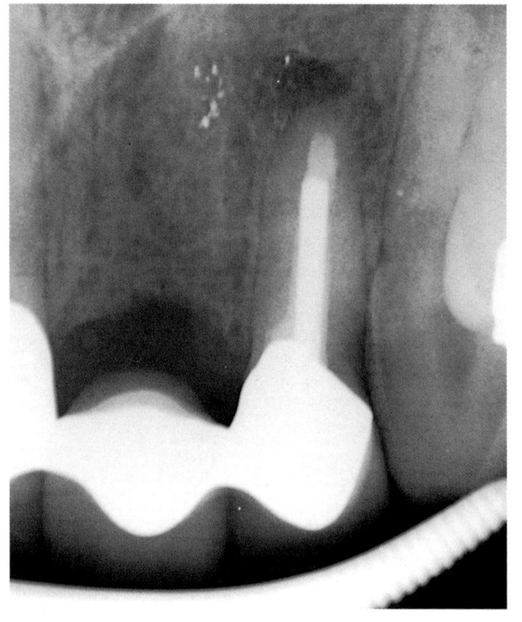

- Radiograph showing *IRM* in situ.

Apical Isolation

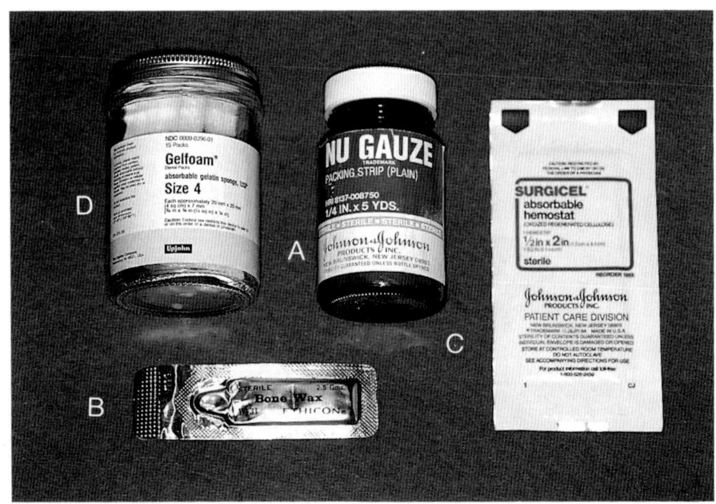

- Hemorrhage control:
  - **A**, *Nu Gauze*
  - **B**, bone wax
  - **C**, *Surgicel*
  - **D**, *Gelfoam*

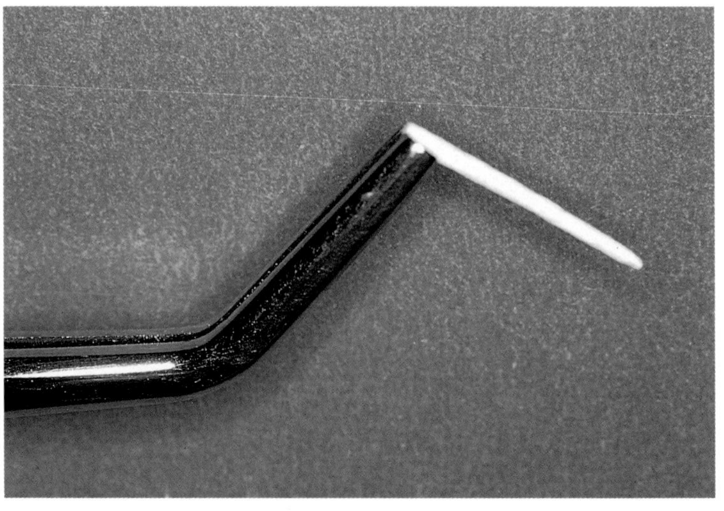

- Drying apical preparation:
  - modified paper points

Visual Magnification

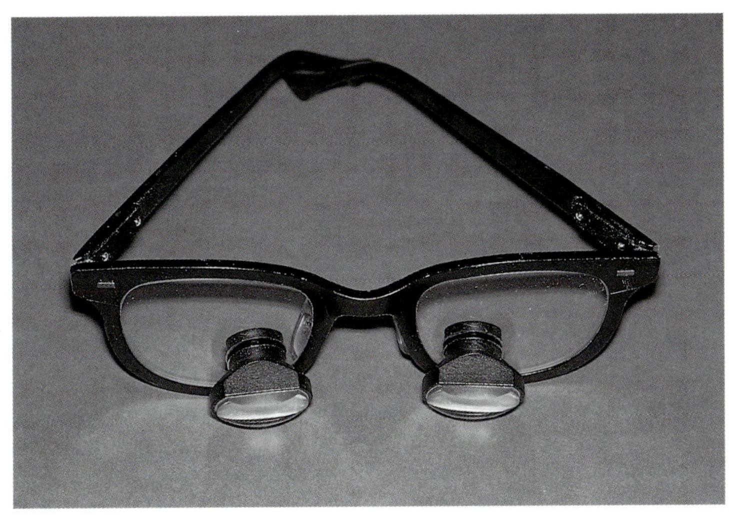

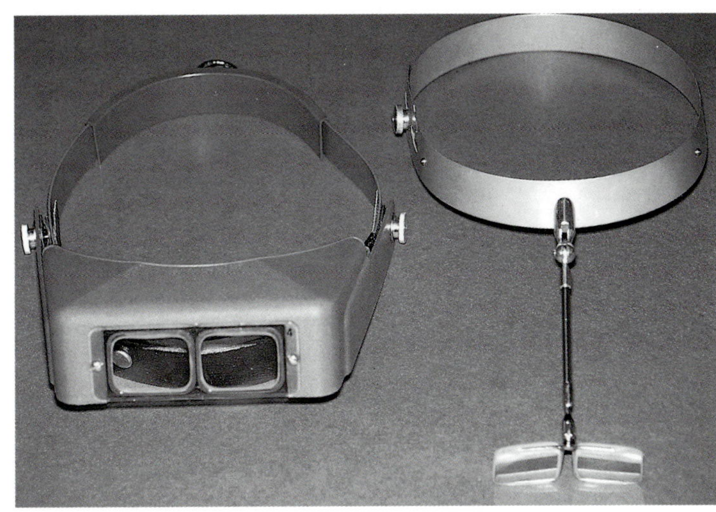

- Enhances visual acuity for detailed precision therapy.
- Facilitates detection of:
  - root fractures
  - perforations
  - inadequate apical seals
  - additional canals
  - root end anomalies

Oral Hygiene

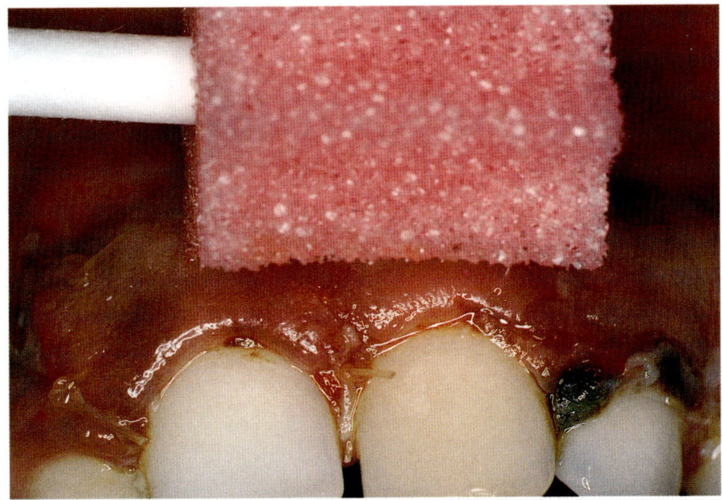

- Disposable toothbrush *(Toothette):*
  - dentifrice impregnated
  - activated by saliva
  - soft and easy to maneuver

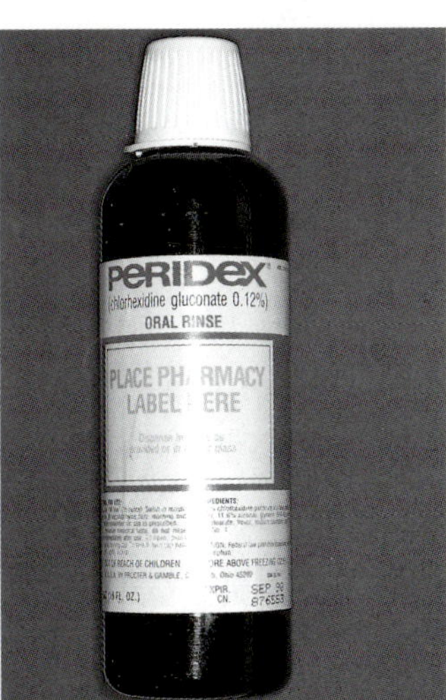

- Chlorhexidine rinse *(Peridex):*
  - as a presurgical rinse, use the day before surgery
  - as a postsurgical rinse, use for 3 to 5 days after surgery

3 Flap Design

Gaining access to the surgical site involves handling tissue that must be incised, reflected, held in position, repositioned, and then sutured to place. Unless these procedures are thought out and followed with sound surgical judgment, the end result can be compromised.

Attention must be directed to the size and shape of the lesion, root length, anatomic landmarks, bony contours, amount of attached gingiva, and presence of prosthetic crown coverage.

Several basic key points in flap design must always be considered. The incision must penetrate through the mucosa and periosteum to the cortical bone. A broad base is required to ensure sufficient blood flow to the flap. The reflection must be atraumatic and include the periosteum. The gingival margins must be carefully incised intrasulcularly, and the interproximal papilla must be freed before reflection. This prevents tearing of the tissue, perforation of the marginal gingiva, and crushing of the interseptal bone.

Access and visibility to the surgical site can be improved by following the basic principles of flap design. In addition, repositioning and suturing of the flap is facilitated.

The basic flap designs used in endodontic surgery currently are:

Gingival	Ochsenbein-Luebke
Semilunar	Rectangular
Triangular	Trapezoidal

Gingival Flap

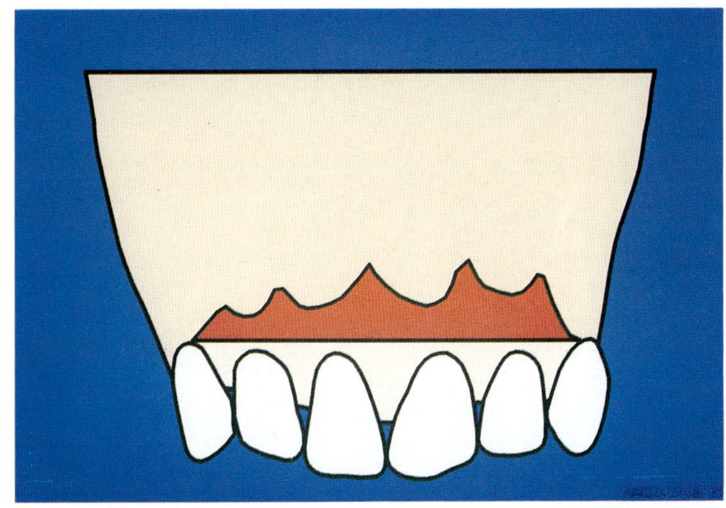

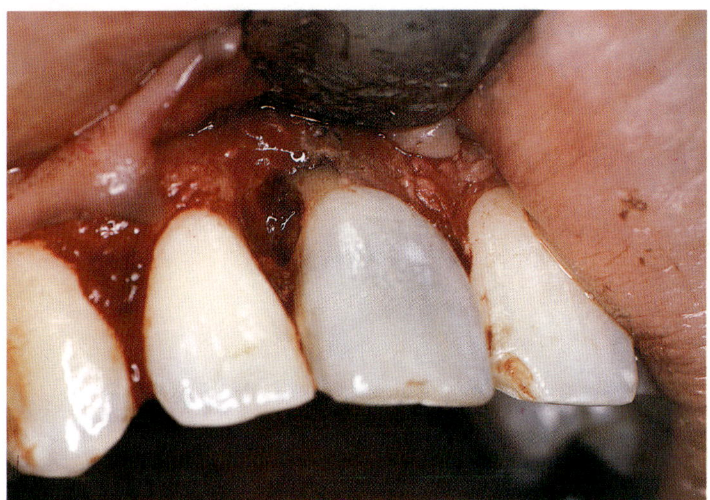

Indications

- Cervical resorptive defects.
- Cervical area perforations.
- Periodontal procedures.

Advantages

- No vertical incision.
- Ease of repositioning.

Disadvantages

- Limited access and visibility.
- Difficult to reflect and retract.
- Predisposed to stretching and tearing.
- Gingival attachment violated.

Surgical technique notes

Vertical incision

The incision should be continuous, linear, and well defined. Avoid repeated incisions through the same tract. Do not make an incision on an eminence or on a pronounced anatomical contour.

The vertical incision should extend from the line angle of the tooth to a length that provides adequate reflection but does not impinge on muscle attachment or highly vascular areas.

It is an accepted standard currently in use to angle the vertical incision to establish a broad base. However, when this is done, impingement on pronounced bony contours occurs and results in suturing under tension. Also, these incisions intrude deeper into soft tissue and usually increase the chance of bleeding, swelling, and postoperative pain. This same broad base can be created when vertical incisions are placed one or two more teeth laterally, thus achieving the same effect. This technique has the added value of reducing the possibility that the flap will be stretched, torn, or sutured under tension. At the same time, it provides a broad base with an adequate blood supply.

Intrasulcular incision

The horizontal incision follows the contours of the labial surfaces of the teeth, dipping interproximally and producing well-defined incisions that effortlessly free the gingival margins.

Semilunar Flap

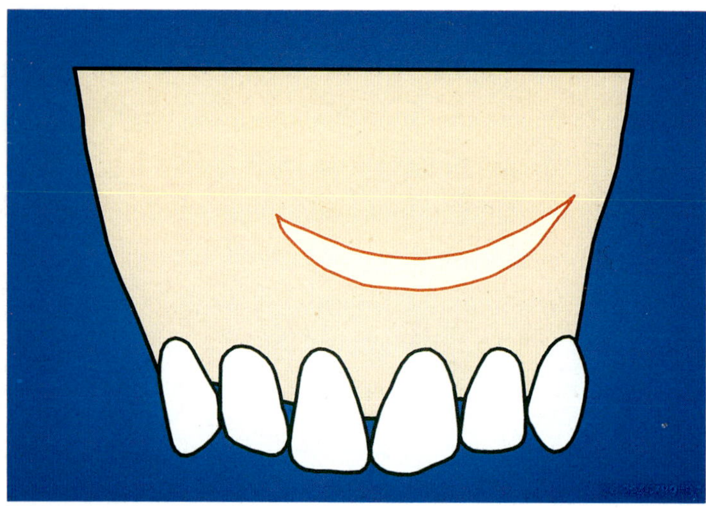

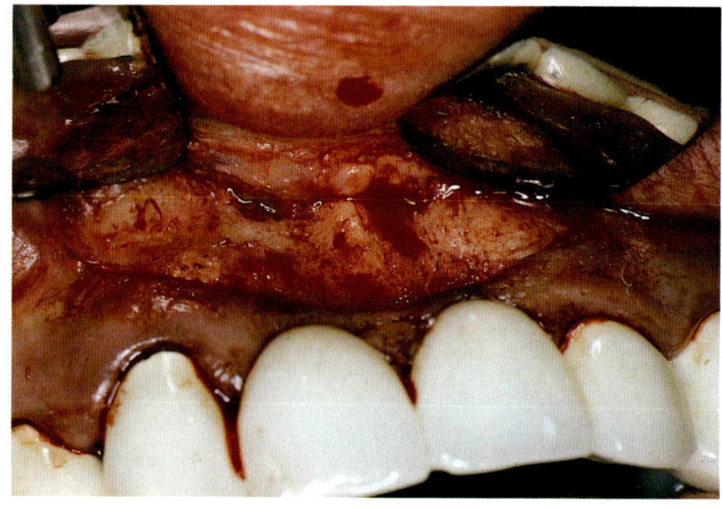

Indications

- Esthetic crowns present.
- Trephination.

Advantages

- Reduces incision and reflection time.
- Maintains integrity of gingival attachment.
- Eliminates potential crestal bone loss.

Disadvantages

- Limited access and visibility.
- Tendency for increased hemorrhaging.
- Crosses root eminences.
- May not include entire lesion.
- Predisposed to stretching and tearing.
- Repositioning is difficult.
- Healing is associated with scarring.

Reflection

Reflection is initiated in the midportion of the vertical incision. The sharp convex end of a no. 4 Molt curet is used to reflect both the periosteum and overlying mucosa; it avoids the crushing pressure on the interproximal crestal bone that frequently occurs when the pointed end of the periosteal elevator is used interproximally to release the marginal gingiva. The flattened, wide end of the periosteal elevator can also be used, even though it is considerably larger and bulkier than the no. 4 Molt curet. The smaller no. 2 Molt curet can also be used to reflect the interproximal tissue, preventing pressure from being exerted on the interseptal bone.

Bony contours

Exercise caution during reflection in areas where there is prominent bony architecture, namely, buttressed bone and bony eminences. Reflection under these conditions could tear and perforate the flap. A quartered 2 x 2 gauze held firmly against the flap acts as a support and facilitates a controlled reflection, which reduces the chances of perforation.

Retractor placement

An aspect of flap reflection that often escapes attention is the placement of the retractor. The retractor should always be placed firmly on bone above the bony defect.

Triangular Flap

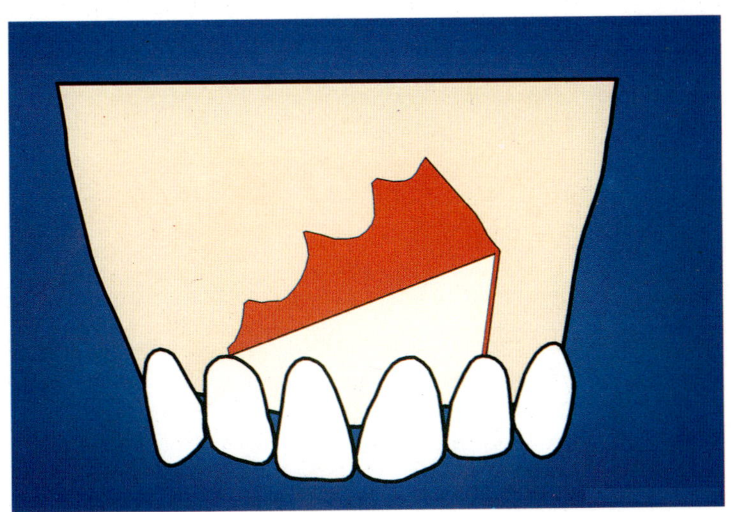

Indications

- Midroot perforation repair.
- Periapical surgery:
  - posterior areas
  - short roots

Advantages

- Easily modified:
  - small relaxing incision
  - additional vertical incision
  - extension of horizontal component
- Easily repositioned.
- Maintains integrity of blood supply.

Disadvantages

- Limited access and visibility to long roots.
- Tension is created on retraction.
- Vertical incision penetrates alveolar mucosa.
- Gingival attachment severed.

Ochsenbein-Luebke Flap

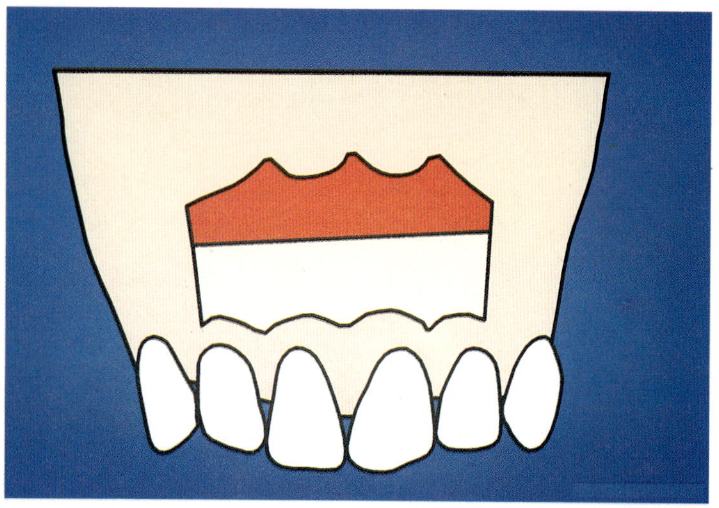

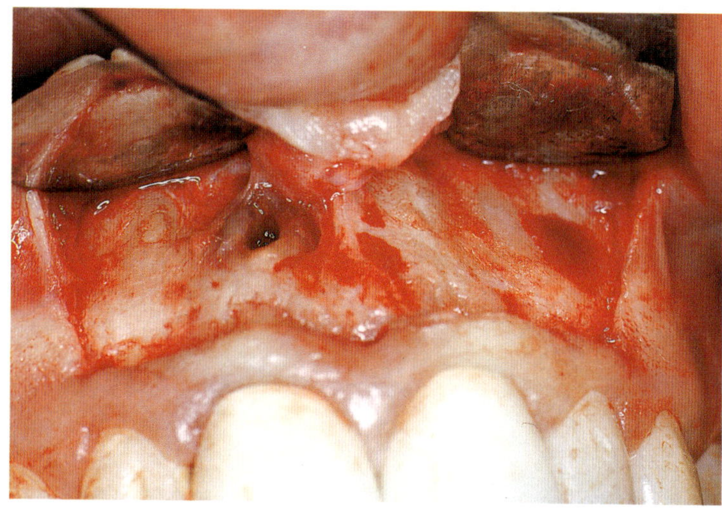

Indications

- Prosthetic crowns present.
- Periapical surgery:
  - —anterior region
  - —longer roots
- Wide band of attached gingiva.

Advantages

- Ease in incision and reflection.
- Enhanced visibility and access.
- Ease in repositioning.
- Maintains integrity of gingival attachment:
  - —prevents gingival recession
  - —avoids dehiscences
  - —prevents crestal bone loss

Disadvantages

- Horizontal component disrupts blood supply.
- Vertical component crosses mucogingival junction and may enter muscle tissue.
- Difficult to alter if size of lesion misjudged.

The reflected tissue should lie freely against the retractor and not be pushed or pulled against the lip or cheek. Always check to confirm that the marginal gingiva and interproximal papilla are not crushed or folded during retraction. The papilla, under these conditions, will become swollen and discolored, which will compromise repositioning, suturing, and healing. Repeated adjustment or repositioning of the retractor may be required during surgical procedures. The exposed bone and flap should be irrigated with normal sterile saline throughout the entire procedure. This will be time well spent.

Closure

Before closure and suturing, copiously irrigate under the flap and over the surrounding bone. The surgical site should be free of any debris or bone fragments. Remove any hemostatic barrier (eg, *Nu Gauze,* bone wax) at this time. Always take a final radiograph before the tissue is repositioned and sutured.

Rectangular Flap

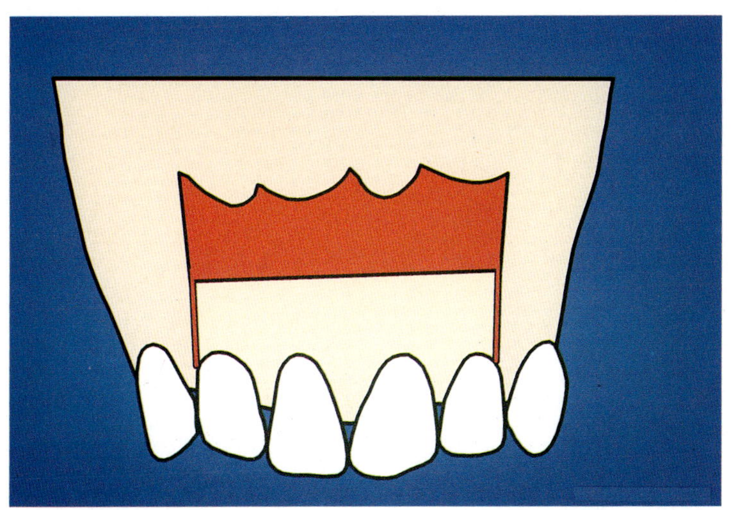

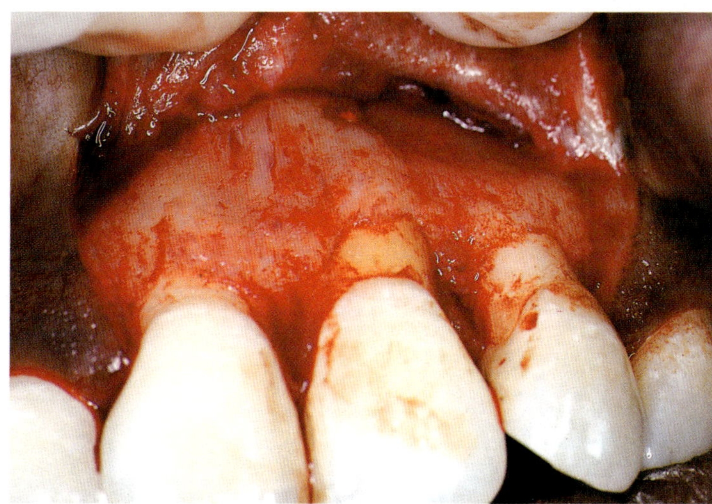

Indications

- Periapical surgery:
  - —multiple teeth
  - —large lesions
  - —long or short roots
- Lateral root repairs:
  - —full-length root visualized

Advantages

- Provides maximum access and visibility.
- Reduces retraction tension.
- Facilitates repositioning.

Disadvantages

- Reduced blood supply to flap.
- Increased incision and reflection time.
- Gingival attachment violated:
  - —gingival recession
  - —crestal bone loss
  - —may uncover dehiscence
- Suturing is more difficult.

4 Suturing

A simple suturing technique commonly used in endodontic surgery involves interrupted sutures placed interproximally and along the vertical component. The technique described in this atlas uses interrupted sutures as well as a single suspensory sling suture around the surgically involved tooth. The suture technique is simple, easy to master, and adaptable to either silk or gut.

The purpose of suturing is to approximate the tissues, provide strength to the wound, and eliminate tissue spaces within the wound. There are many types of sutures to choose from and several suturing techniques. However, they all achieve the same result.

Failed sutures are usually caused by certain factors. Poor knot security and placement result in torn and separated sutures. Excessive tension may lead to incision juxtaposition and inappropriate alignment. Failure to eliminate tissue spaces may result in the pooling of blood and hematoma formation, which produces pain and swelling.

Absorbable gut is referred to as *catgut.* It is manufactured from collagen obtained from the small intestine of sheep or cattle. When untreated it is called *plain gut. Chromic gut* is treated with chromic salts to provide greater resistance to absorption, but it is not routinely used in endodontic surgery. Silk sutures are made from the protein-rich thread spun by silkworm larvae while making their cocoons.

Several advantages of silk sutures are their visibility, knot security, and ease in knotting. Among the disadvantages of silk is its "wicking" action of tissue fluids and bacteria. It also has a tendency to promote plaque formation and induce a greater inflammatory response.

Many clinicians prefer plain gut sutures because there is no removal time involved or painful postsurgical removal. It is also convenient for those patients who are unable to return for regular postsurgical followup. The absorption of these sutures is related to enzyme activity and the acidity of the oral cavity. Like silk, gut sutures should always be hydrated before use; this will facilitate manipulation and reduce tissue drag. Although gut sutures have been said to demonstrate poor manipulative properties and knot security, this has not been borne out by experienced clinicians. A major drawback is its visibility. The sutures tend to blend in with the background because they are translucent. Gut, like silk, when used in the 4-0 filament thread size with a conventional cutting needle, is ideally suited for endodontic needs.

The clinician can choose from three different instruments when suturing: a hemostat, needle holder, or mosquito forceps. Needle holders are ideal for reaching deep into the recesses of the oral cavity. The longer handle also gives a degree of measured control frequently required. The needle holder used together with a half-circled swaged needle can easily rotate through tissue in the most limited confines of the oral cavity.

Surgical technique notes

Suture selection

Either 4-0 silk or absorbable gut, used with a half-circled swaged needle, is the suture material of choice for almost all surgical endodontic procedures. Selection is based on the advantages and disadvantages previously mentioned and in many cases is clinician-dependent.

Suture technique

Grasp the needle away from the tip and below the swaged end, about midpoint; engaging the needle at the tip dulls the cutting edge and can bend it out of shape, which can result in cutting and tearing of the delicate tissue. When held at the swaged end, the needle can become distorted, thus interrupting passage through tissue and the interproximal spaces.

Readapt the tissue and hold it under light pressure several minutes before suturing. Complete the single sling suspensory suture first; it adapts the tissue firmly around the tooth in question. Then place interrupted sutures at the appropriate intervals to secure the flap. Tissue is always sutured from the unattached surface of the mucosa to an attached surface of the mucosa. Frequently, vertical sutures are not necessary if alignment and approximation have been done with care. However, if vertical sutures are required, they should be adequately spaced and used only where necessary. Complete the final tie with a surgeon's knot. When making the tie, clinicians frequently pull up on the suture, thereby elevating the tissue from the bone and disrupting the fibrin clot. When making the final tie, direct the pressure toward the tissue and avoid elevating the flap. At this point, many clinicians prefer a hand tie to ensure control and a snug readaptation of both overlying tissue and the suture. Avoid placing knots over the incision line. Also, avoid cutting the suture too close to the knot to prevent unravelling.

Suturing over an eminence or irregular bony contour can impede the needle from engaging the tissue along the incision line. When this occurs, the tissue is placed under tension, the blood supply is compromised, and tearing of the suture is a certainty. Suturing so tightly that the tissue becomes ischemic results in torn sutures and/or sloughed tissue.

Suture removal

Nonabsorbable sutures are usually maintained in site for 3 to 5 days, whereas absorbable sutures show signs of dissolution in about 3 to 7 days. Occasionally, knots from absorbable sutures remain longer because they are bulky.

Single Suspensory and Interrupted Suturing Technique

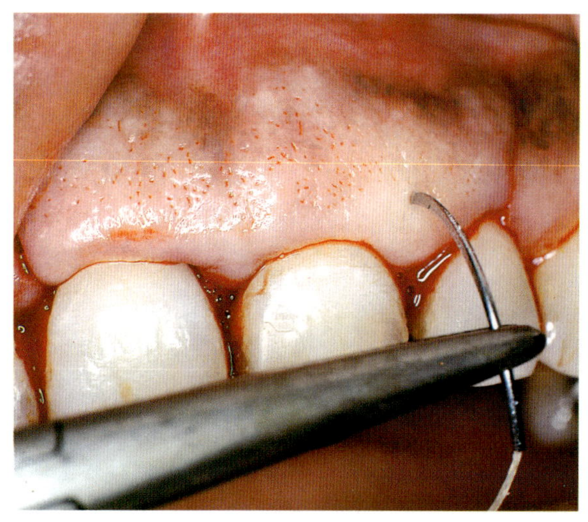

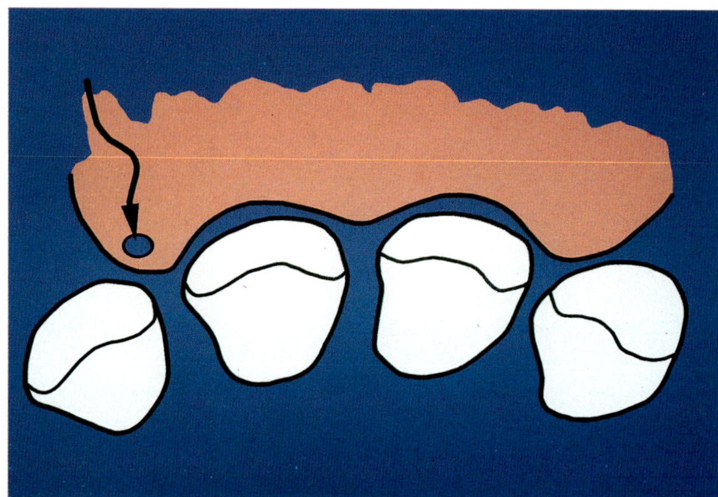

- Begin suspensory suture on surgically involved tooth.
- Engage unattached flap on facial surface.

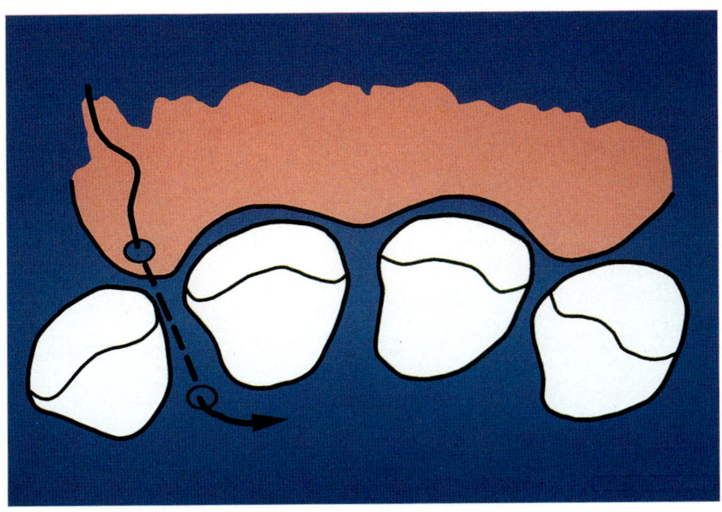

• Continue interproximally engaging the inferior surface of the attached lingual tissue.

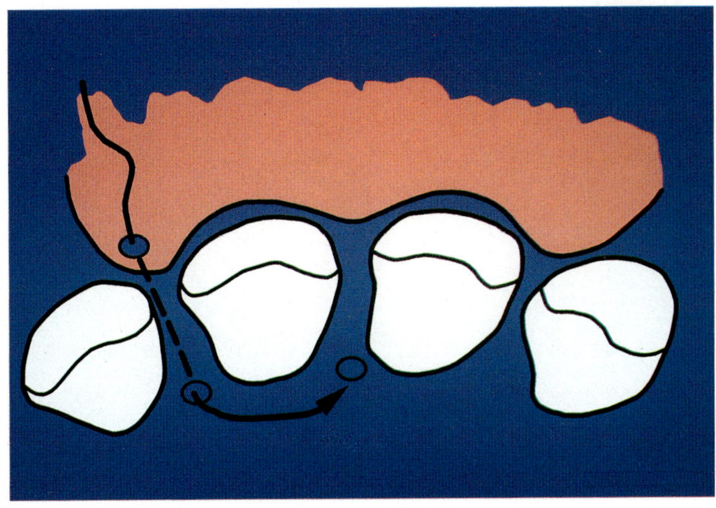

• Encircle the lingual aspect of the tooth and engage lingual tissue.

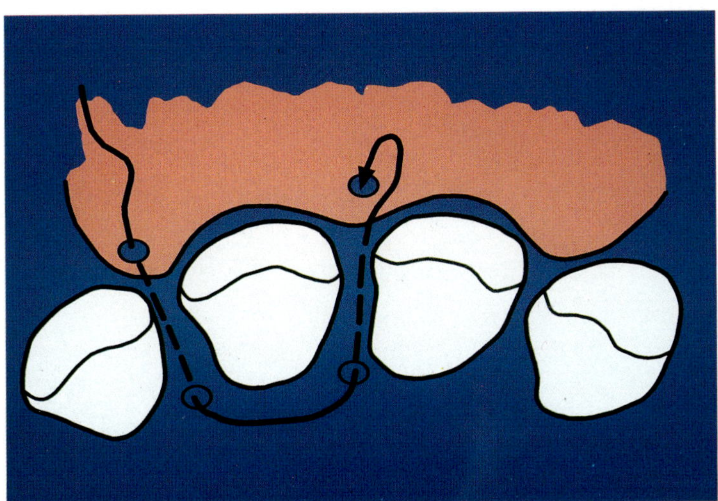

• Pass suture interproximally without engaging undersurface of flap.

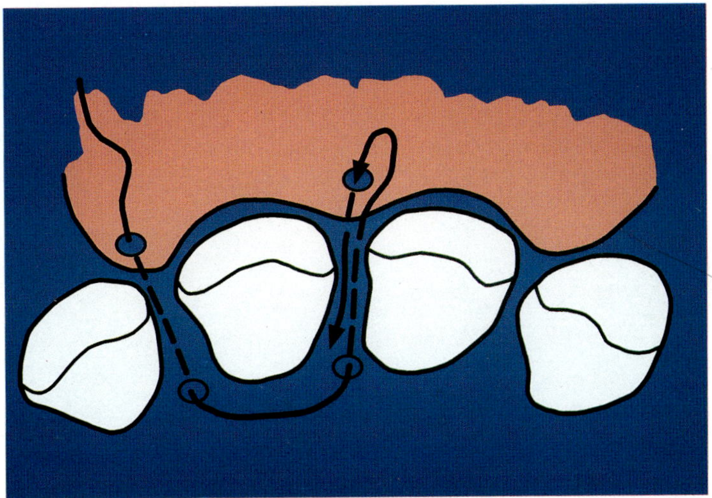

• Insert needle through unattached flap on facial surface and pass interproximally.

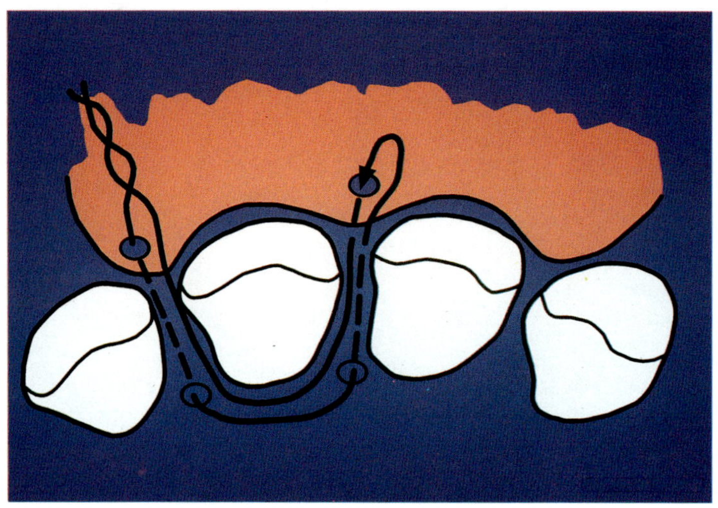

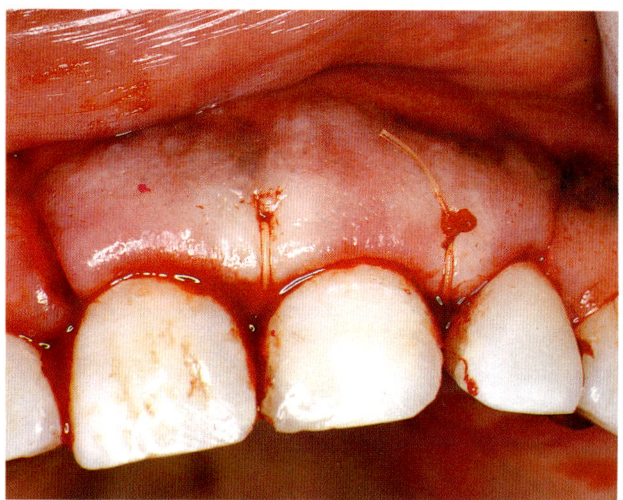

- Wrap suture around lingual surface.
- Pass interproximally without tissue engagement.
- Tie knot at initial entry point.

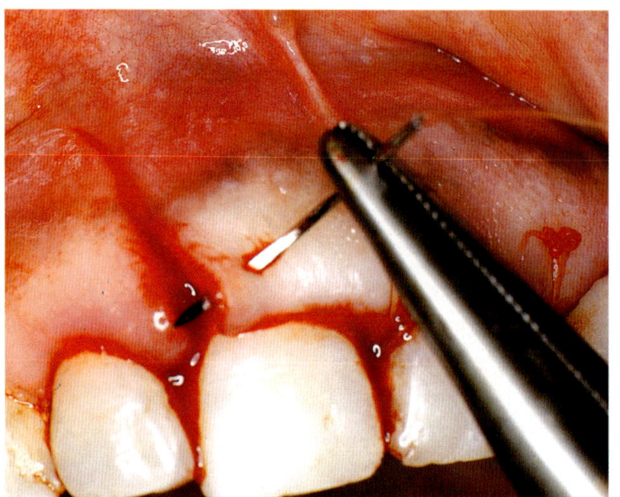

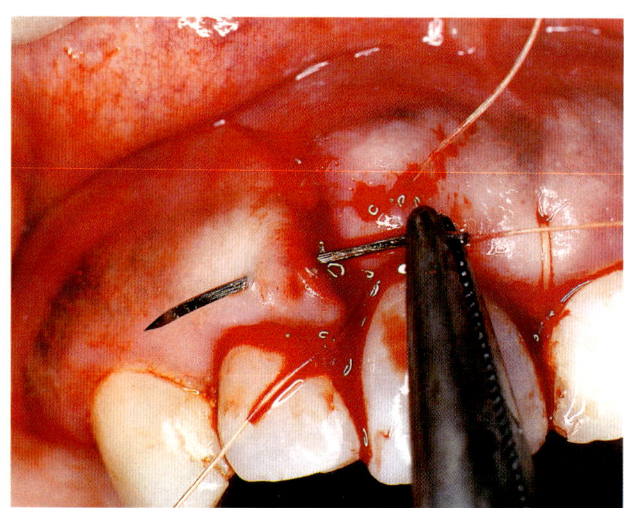

- Place interrupted sutures interproximally and along vertical incisions as required for closure.

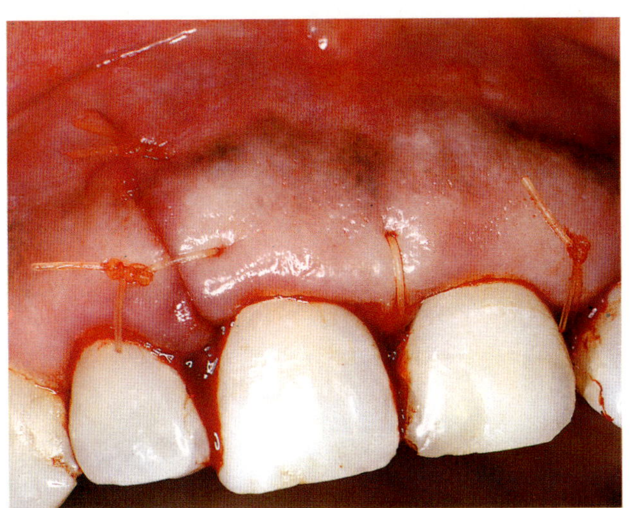

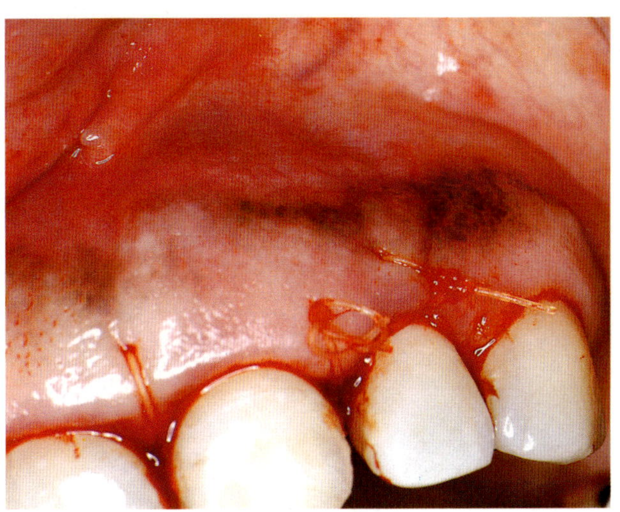

- Completed closure consists of a single suspensory suture with accompanying interrupted sutures.

5 Incision and Drainage

Fluctuant soft tissue swellings occur when periapical inflammatory exudate flows through the medullary bone and eventually perforates the cortical plate. Once through the cortical plate, the exudate lifts up and separates the periosteum, spreading into the surrounding soft tissue. When this occurs, incision and drainage are the surgical techniques used to reduce the swelling and render relief. As most clinicians will assert, the timing of incision and drainage has always been tempered by the patient's signs and symptoms and the clinician's experience.

Vestibular swellings that are fluctuant and localized are ideal candidates for incision and drainage. Caution should always be exercised where swellings are generalized, diffuse, and/or indurated, especially when accompanied with associated fever and extension of the swelling into fascial planes and anatomic spaces. A cellulitis of this nature can be life-threatening, for which a combined effort of culturing, antibiotic therapy, hospitalization, and additional consultation may be required. A baseline temperature and description of the swelling is always noted in the record before any surgical procedure is undertaken.

Surgical technique notes

Basic incision and drainage tray setup

The organization and tray layout should reflect simplicity and minimize clutter. Instruments should be laid out in the order of treatment sequence.

Anesthesia

Block injection is considered the ideal method of obtaining complete anesthesia prior to incision and drainage. In some localized areas a combination of block anesthesia and local infiltration complement each other in ensuring profound anesthesia and reduced patient anxiety. A topical anesthetic is placed over the center of the fluctuant mass, followed by a subcutaneous infiltration that blanches the superficial tissue. When this occurs, the swelling is ready to be incised and drained.

Drain selection and preparation

The main objective is to keep the surgical site patent and allow for continuous drainage, which is accomplished by a mechanical drain. Sterile rubber dam has historically served this purpose; however, its size, various shapes, and lack of bulk as well as ease of displacement are noteworthy drawbacks. An alternative that is more functional and biologically sound is a ¼-inch *Penrose* drain. Drain length depends on the size of the lesion and depth of placement. The lateral borders of the *Penrose* drain are serrated for mechanical retention and act as additional vents, enhancing drainage.

Culture and sensitivity

A sterile syringe can be used to aspirate the swelling. The aspirant is sealed and forwarded to the laboratory for culturing and sensitivity testing. An alternative technique is to sample the drainage discharge after the incision is made. The material is then placed in a specially designed packet and sent to the laboratory. Regardless of which technique is used, both aerobic and anaerobic detection techniques should always be requested. Laboratory processing should be accomplished as soon as possible.

Incision and drainage

Direct a no. 11 blade through the fluctuant mass perpendicular to the bone and through the periosteum. In most cases a vertical incision is made; however, a horizontal incision may be necessary in cases of broad swellings. Avoid misdirected incisions into soft tissue and muscle. Exercise caution when incising near anatomic landmarks (eg, mental foramen and greater palatine neurovascular bundle) to prevent unnecessary swelling, bleeding, pain, and possibly an additional path for the spread of the infection. Once the fluctuant area has been penetrated, drainage usually follows unimpeded.

Blunt dissection

Blunt dissection is referred to as "spreading" of the incision after initial drainage. Insert a small curved *Kelly* hemostat into the incision site and direct it laterally and vertically. Open the hemostat gently during the probing action to penetrate and disrupt any pockets or recesses of purulent material not already released as a result of the initial incision and drainage. The depth of penetration during spreading also facilitates drain placement and ensures adequate drain depth.

Irrigation

Before the drain is placed, the incision and drainage site is irrigated copiously with sterile saline. This lavage action flushes out the remaining exudate and/or clotted blood, which might act to impede drain placement.

Drain placement

Secure the previously prepared drain to the mucosa by means of a 4-0 silk suture. Place it into position with the curved *Kelly* hemostat and insert with gentle pressure until it is firmly seated within the incision site. Check its position and mechanical retention before the overlying tissue is released. Warm saline rinses may be recommended to facilitate drainage and keep the drain patent.

Drain removal

The drain is generally kept in place for 24 to 48 hours, depending on the patient's response to therapy. Remove the drain by releasing the security suture and then easing the drain out. Warm saline rinses are suggested until closure begins and drainage has ceased.

Initial soft tissue healing

The patient should be monitored after drain removal to ensure that the acute condition along with its symptoms have responded to therapy. Note temperature recordings until they register normal. Incision and drainage may not be the definitive treatment. The present condition must be reviewed, the cause established, and the patient treatment planned for definitive therapy.

Basic Incision and Drainage Tray Setup

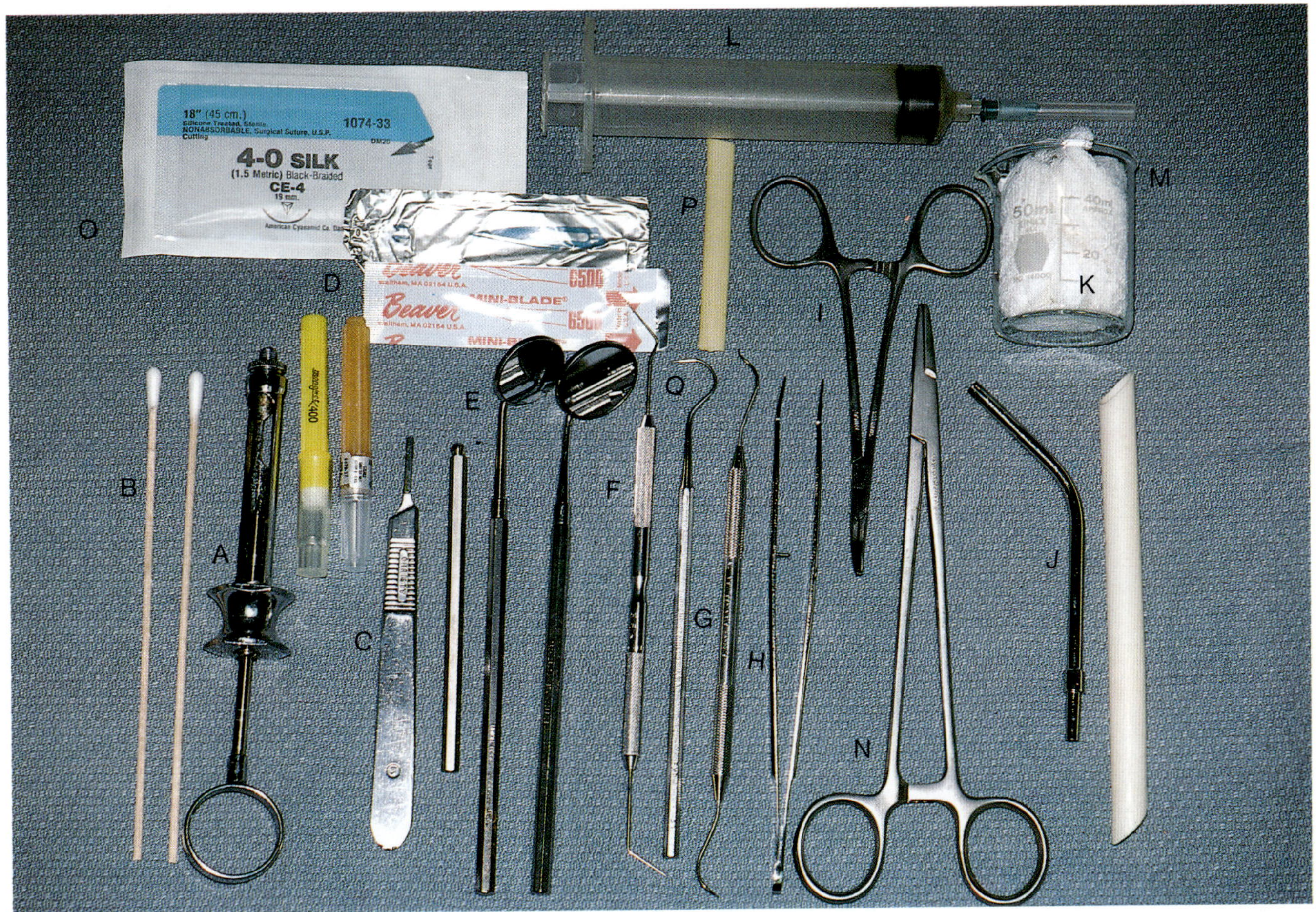

A, Anesthetic syringe and needles; **B,** Cotton-tip applicators; **C,** Surgical blade handle; **D,** Surgical blade (no. 11); **E,** Mirrors; **F,** Endodontic explorer; **G,** Periodontal curet; **H,** Cotton pliers; **I,** Small curved hemostat; **J,** Suction tips (large and small); **K,** Irrigation receptacle; **L,** 20-mL irrigating syringe; **M,** 2 × 2 gauze; **N,** Needle holder; **O,** Suture material (4-0 silk); **P,** ¼-inch *Penrose* drain; **Q,** No. 23 explorer.

Supplemental items not shown: carpules of anesthetic and irrigation solution (sterile saline).

Preoperative Radiographic Examination

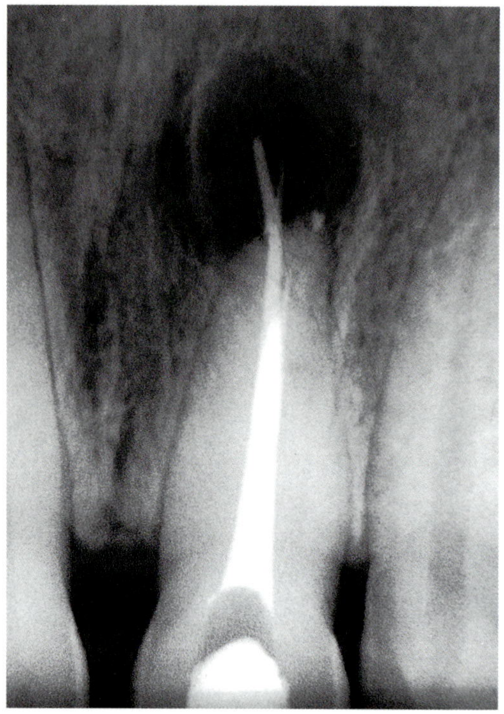

- Acute flare-up subsequent to recent obturation with overextension.
- Periapical radiolucency associated with obturated tooth.

Preoperative Soft Tissue Examination

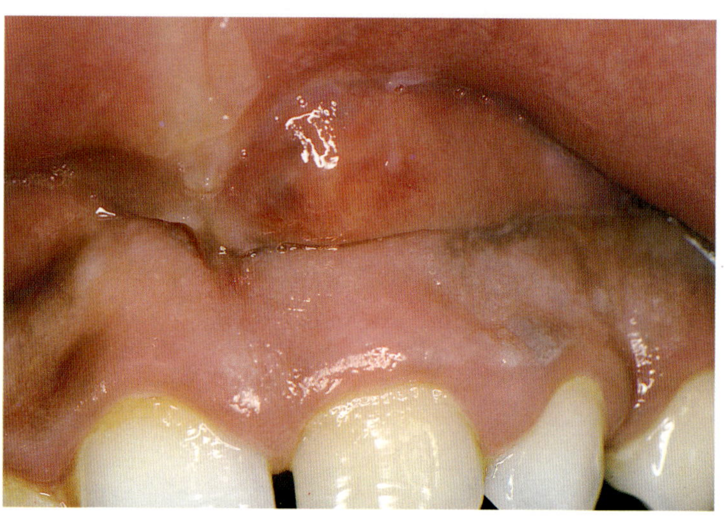

- Localized, fluctuant swelling.
- Patient is afebrile.
- No apparent facial swelling.

Anesthesia

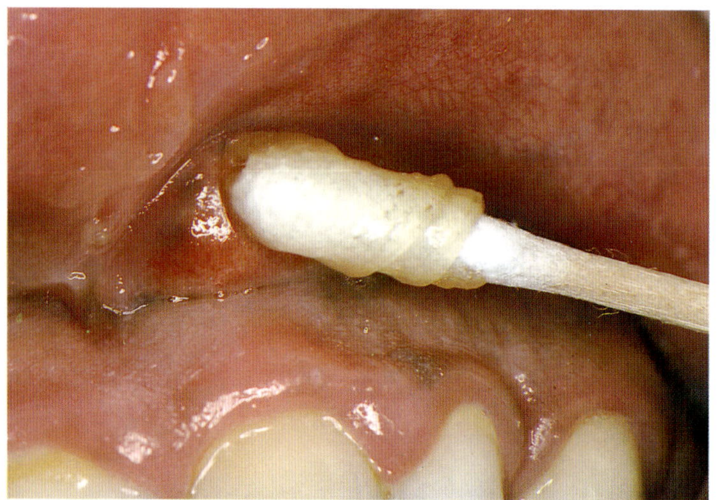

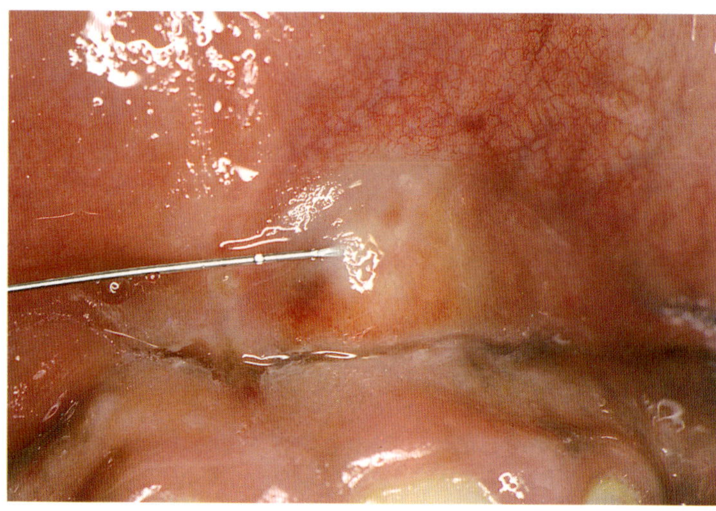

- Localized topical application.
- Subcutaneous injection and blanching.
- Block anesthesia in conjunction with subcutaneous injection.

Incision

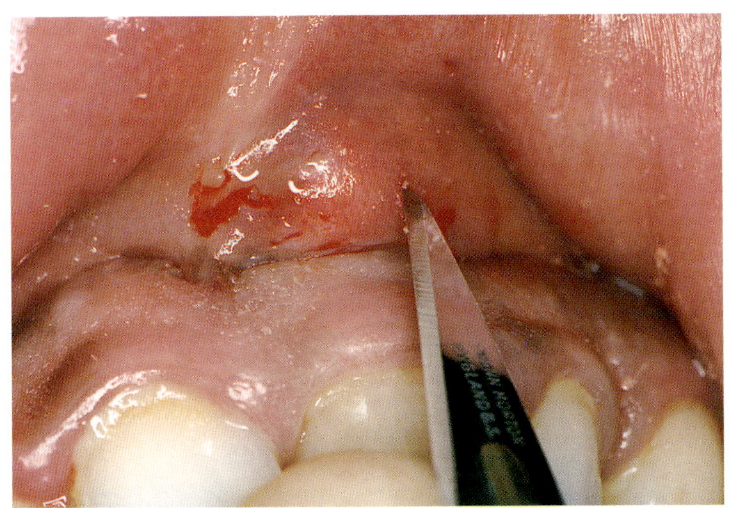

- Use a no. 11 blade.
- Make incision into center of flucuency.

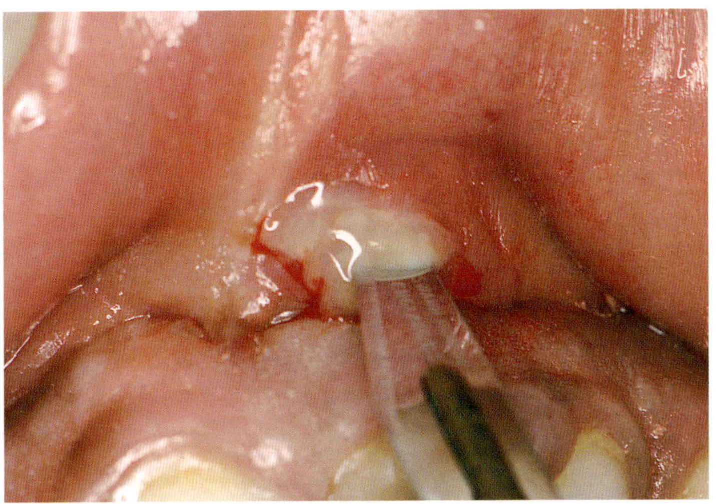

- Make stab incision through soft tissue and periosteum to bone.
- Determine incision length according to dimension of swelling.

Drainage

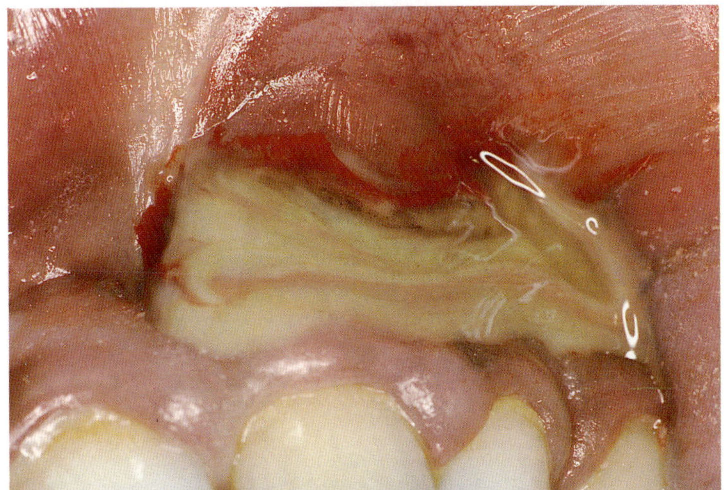

- Initial surgical drainage:
  - purulent
  - sanguinous
- Take culture.

Culture and Sensitivity

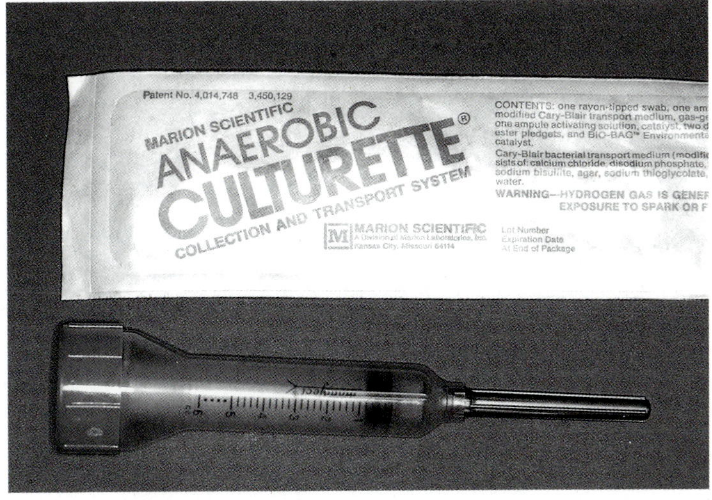

- Materials:
  - *Culturette* (aerobic, anaerobic)
  - needle and syringe for culture aspiration

Blunt Dissection

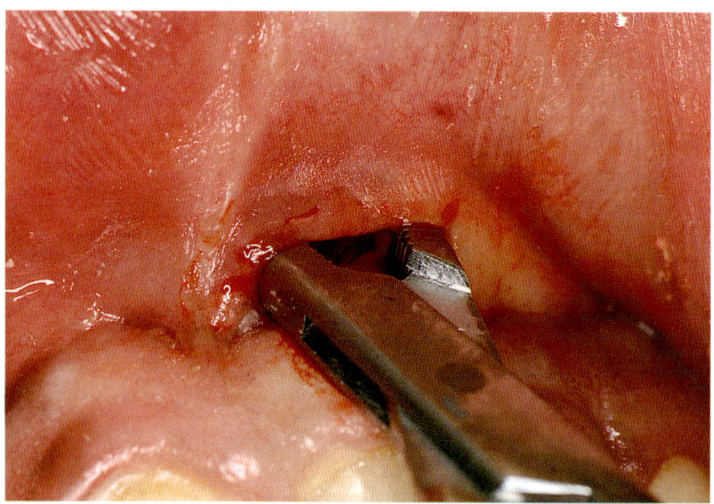

- Explore soft tissue.
- Evacuate recessed purulent pockets.
- Determine drain length according to depth of penetration.

Irrigation

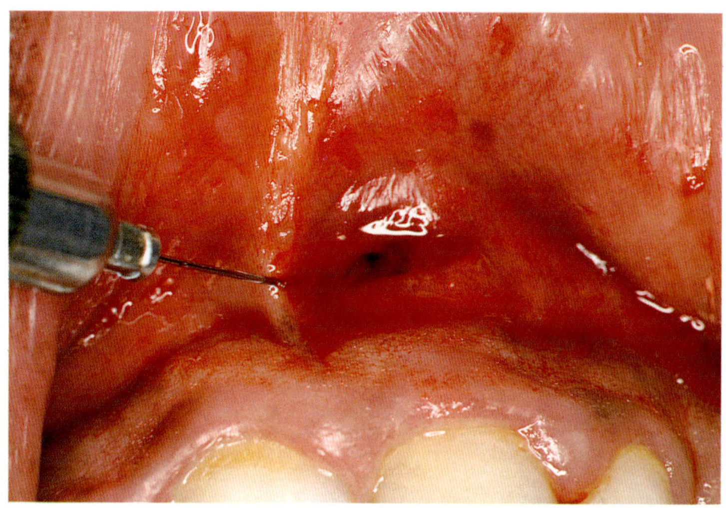

- Solutions:
  — sterile saline
  — sterile anesthetic
- Provides flushing lavage into the lesion.

Drain Preparation

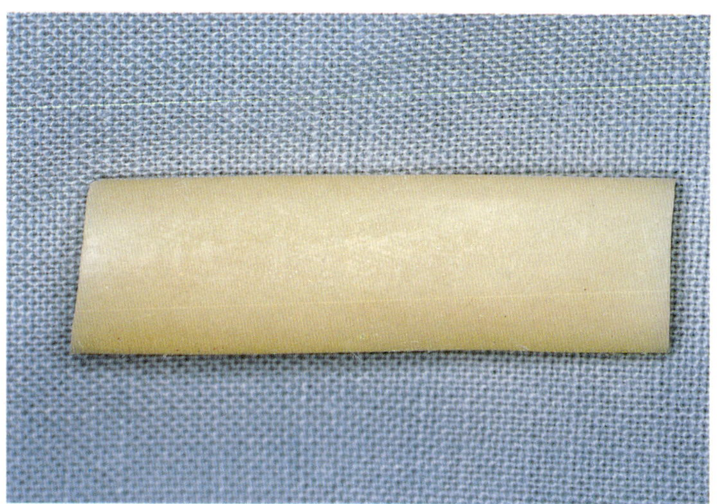

- Penrose drain (¼ inch).

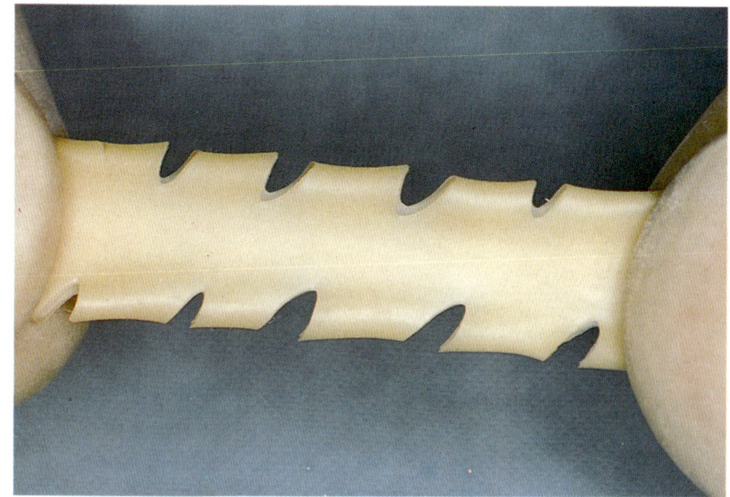

- Serrated edges act as additional drainage vents and provide mechanical retention.

Drain Placement

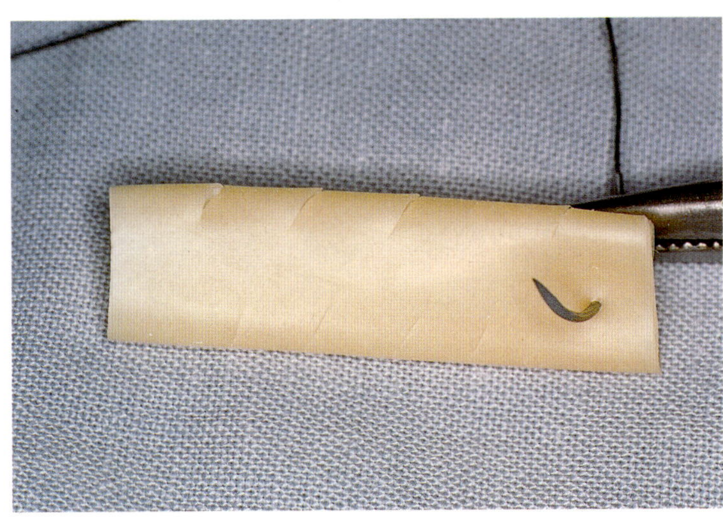

- Secure suture to drain before placing drain into incision.

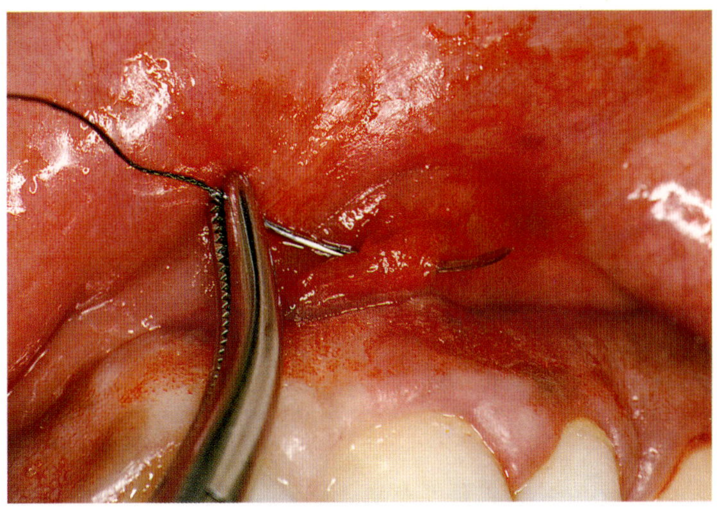

- Secure suture to tissue.

Drain Insertion

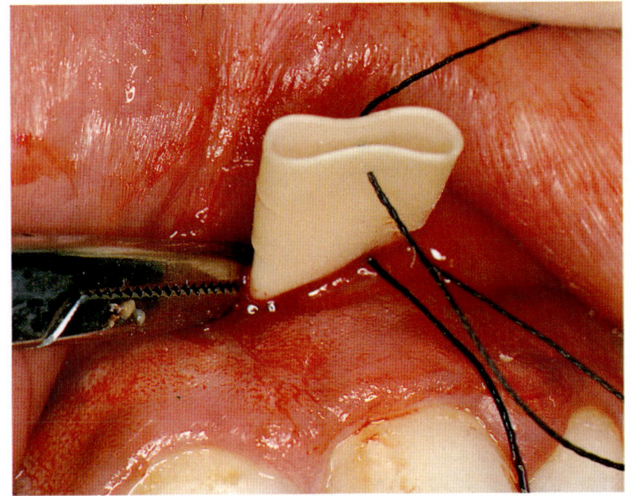

- Insert drain with gentle pressure.
- Use curved *Kelly* hemostat.
- Insert to depth of blunt dissection.

Drain Secured to Tissue

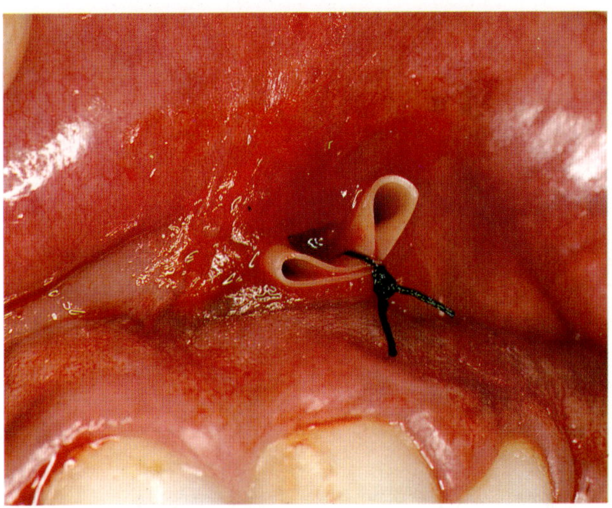

- Check mechanical retention.
- Advise patient to use warm saline rinses to facilitate drainage.

Drain Removal

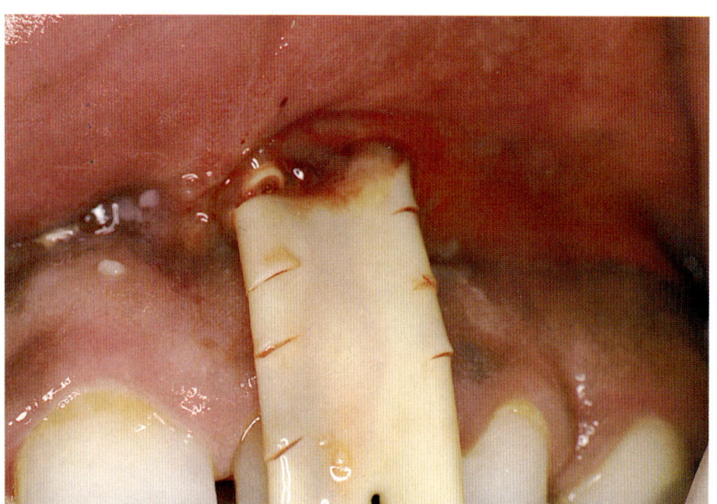

- Remove drain after 24 to 48 hours.
- Timing of drain removal depends on patient's response to therapy.

Initial Soft Tissue Healing

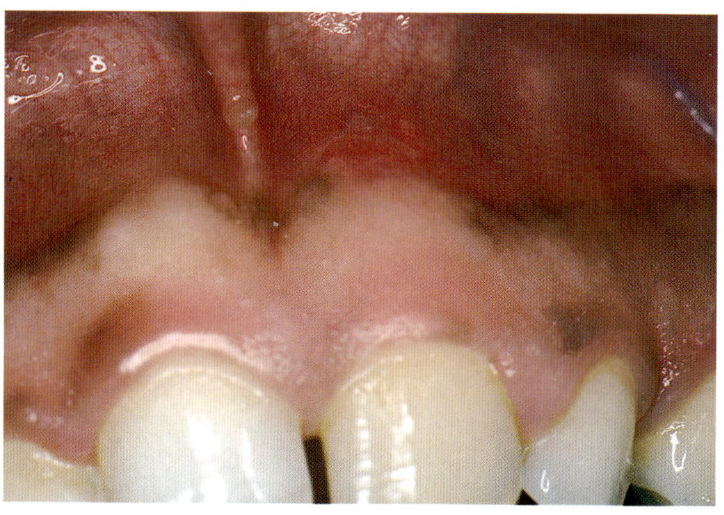

- Monitor patient's response to treatment.
- Schedule appropriate definitive treatment.

Definitive Treatment

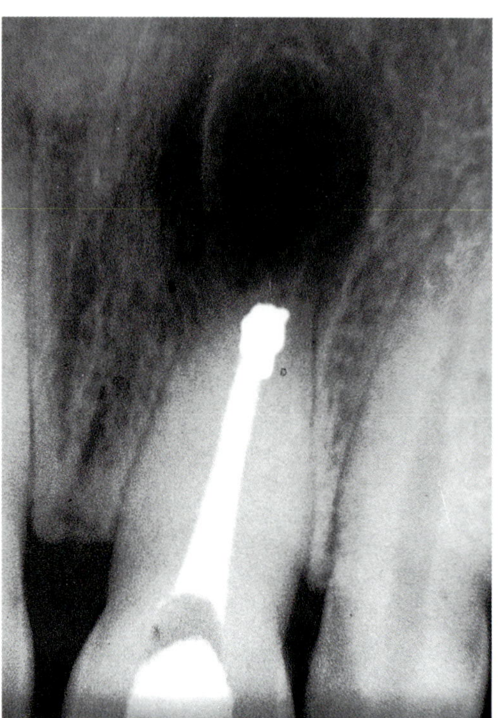

- Surgical enucleation and removal of overextension.
- Root resection.
- Amalgam retrofill.

Six-Month Followup Radiograph

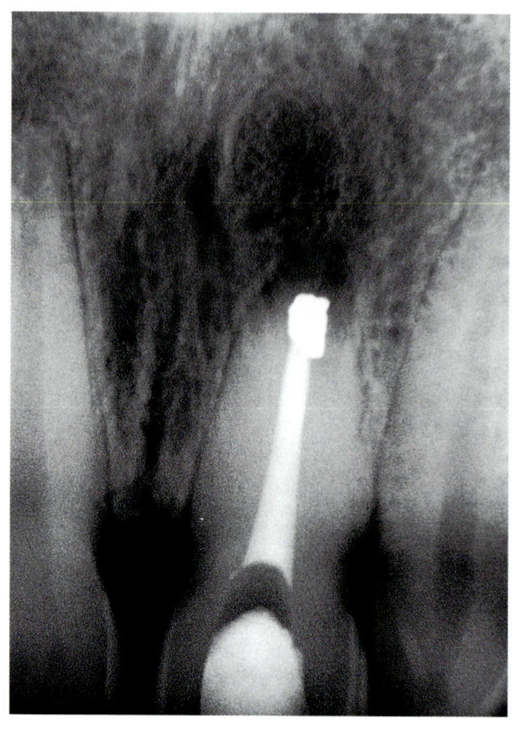

- Patient is asymptomatic.
- Initial osseous repair is evident.

6 Trephination

Trephination is a surgical technique used to alleviate acute pain caused by an accumulation of purulent material when drainage through the root canal is impossible. It involves making an incision through the mucoperiosteum to the alveolar plate of bone over an involved root end. A penetration is made through the bone into the purulent-filled cavity, thereby establishing drainage and relieving the acute symptoms. It is usually performed as an emergency procedure in the absence of soft tissue swelling.

Presurgical technique notes

Presurgical periapical radiograph

The periapical radiograph is used to establish endometrics, detect the presence or absence of a lesion, and determine the lesion size and shape. In addition, relationships of anatomical structures, root angulations, and the status of the root canal (eg, calcifications), the presence of a post, or blockage secondary to previous root canal therapy should be identified.

Endometrics

An estimated measurement of the root length is taken from the radiograph. This measurement can be transferred and superimposed over the tooth in question, indicating the approximate root length and apex location.

Anesthesia

Apply a topical anesthetic locally over the surgical site; this is accompanied by local infiltration. Depending on the location of the lesion, block anesthesia may be required in conjunction with infiltration. Begin the trephination procedure once the proper level of anesthesia is obtained.

Incision

Make a vertical mucoperiosteal incision to cortical bone. Place it as close to the estimated apex as possible, either mesial or distal to it, to avoid damaging the root during trephination. Avoid trephination on any root eminence.

Tissue reflection

Reflect the tissue and expose the cortical bone. Prior to bur preparation inspect the bone for a pathologic fenestration or a weak point, using an endodontic explorer.

Cortical bone penetration

With the tissue reflected and cortical bone visibility assured, penetrate the cortical plate with a round bur of suitable size. Make this apical penetration either to the mesial or distal area of the involved root. It should penetrate through cortical bone and establish drainage. In cases that do not present with a picture of a frank periapical radiolucency, endometrics and apical trephination are done with extreme caution and careful exploration. The absence of a periapical radiolucency does not mean that a purulent area is nonexistent.

Posttreatment followup

Subsequent to initial therapy, the patient is monitored and the course of recovery is followed. Trephination only relieves the symptoms; it is not always a definitive treatment. If trephination does not relieve acute symptoms, or if swelling results and the patient becomes febrile, additional therapy and antibiotic coverage may be required.

Presurgical Periapical Radiograph

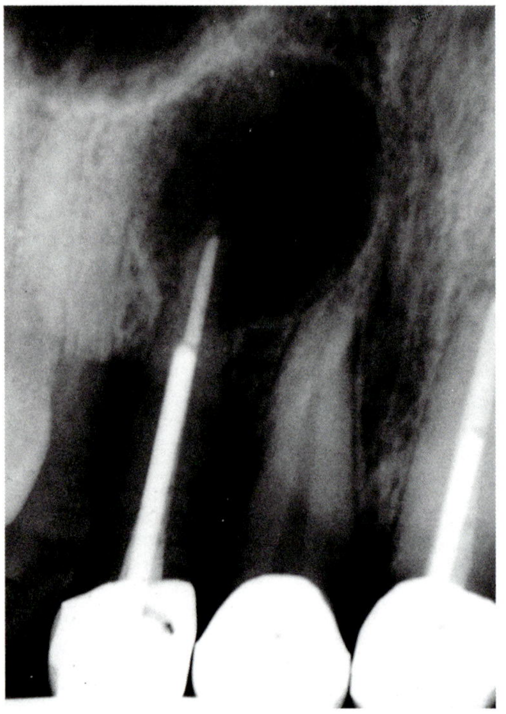

- Inaccessible root canal due to post and crown.
- Periapical radiolucency extends to anterior limit of the maxillary sinus and encroaches on the floor of the nasal cavity.
- Root is straight and parallel to adjacent teeth.
- Root length is determined.

Endometrics

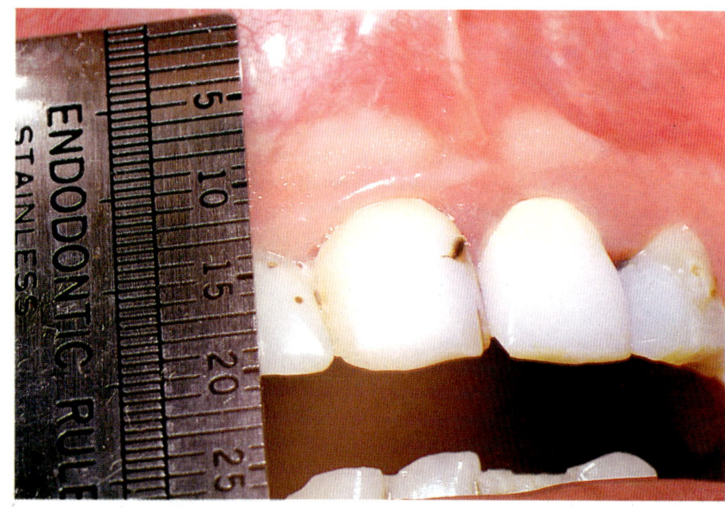

- Approximate position of root apex is determined clinically.
  —soft tissue transfer of radiographic length

Incision Placement

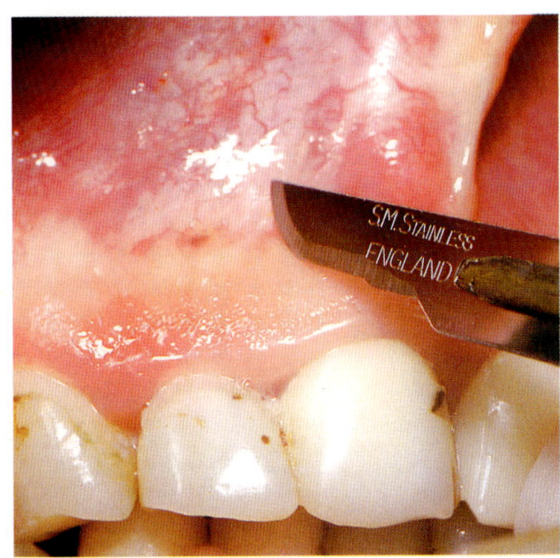

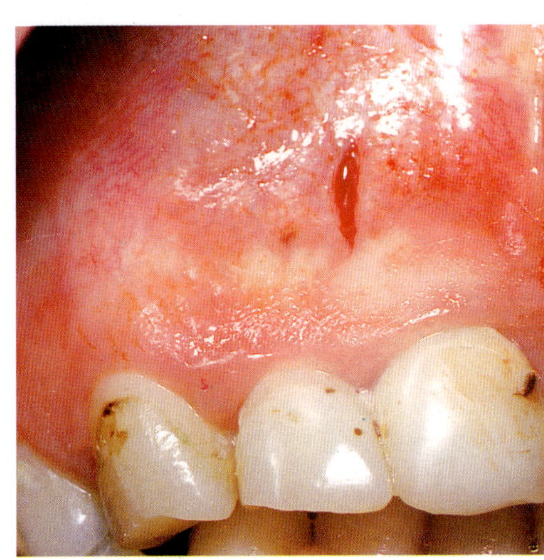

- Vertical incision.
- Placed near approximate position of apex.
- Placed between root eminences.

Exploration of Cortical Bone

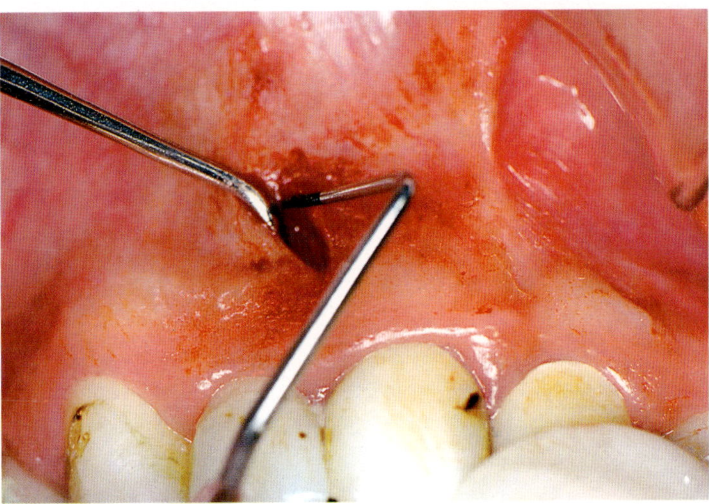

- Intact cortical bone.
- Area of weakened cortical density.
- Pathologic fenestration.

Cortical Bone Penetration

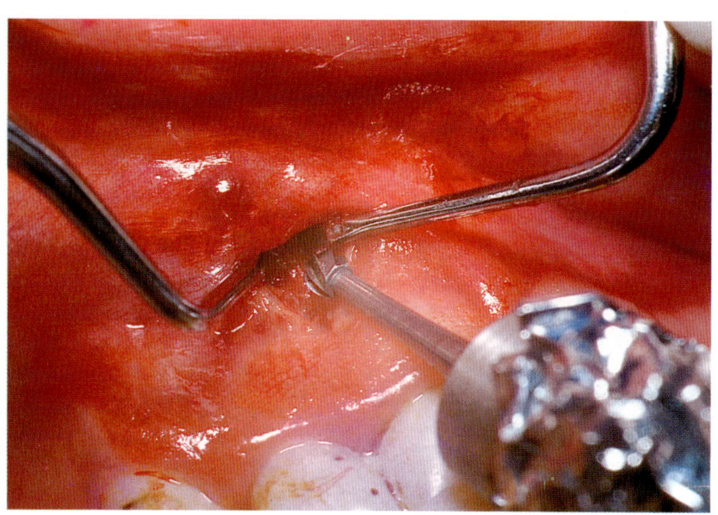

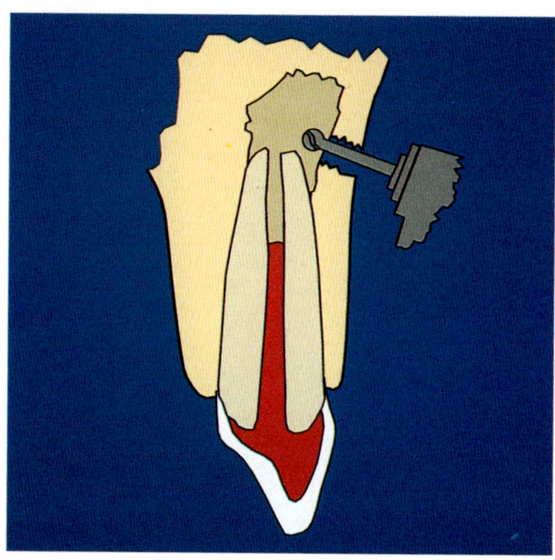

- Directed into center of the lesion.
- Near apex of involved tooth.
- Provides relief of pain and pressure.

Six-Month Radiographic Followup

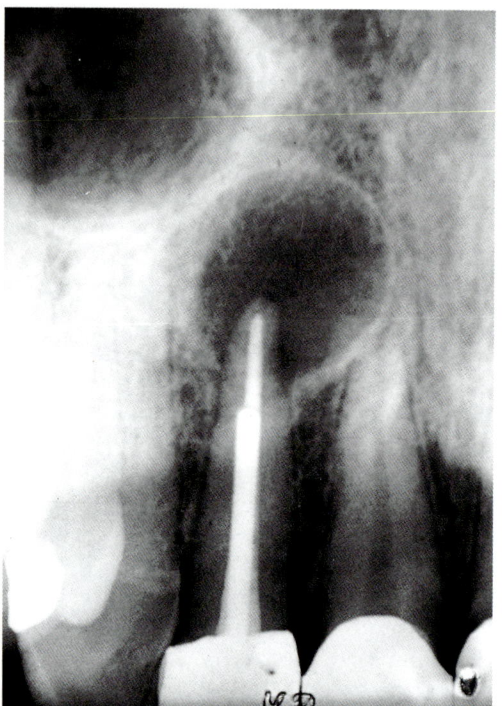

- Lesion decreasing in size.
- Initial osseous repair is evident.

One-Year Radiographic Followup

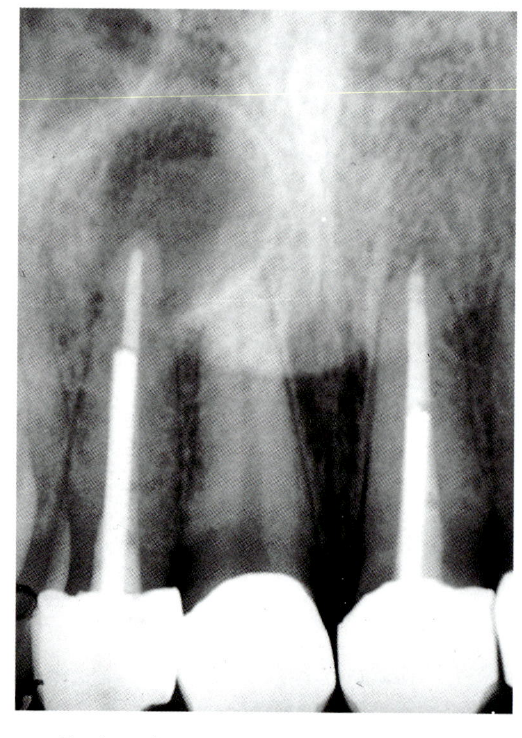

- Patient is asymptomatic.
- Continued osseous repair is evident.

7 Decompression

The effective management of large periapical radiolucent lesions involves consideration of the proximity of the lesion to adjacent vital teeth and encroachment on anatomic structures (eg, maxillary sinus, floor of the nose, mandibular canal, and mental foramen). Successful decompression procedures also depend on patient cooperation, involve lengthy periods of treatment time, and most importantly, depend on the differential diagnosis of the lesion. Many patients present without acute symptoms or facial swellings. Many times these large lesions are discovered on routine examination.

The differential diagnosis of any large periapical lesion must take into consideration the following pathological conditions:

1. Periapical cyst
2. Periapical granuloma
3. Primordial cyst
4. Traumatic bone cyst
5. Aneurysmal bone cyst
6. Central giant cell granuloma
7. Hemangioma
8. Myxoma
9. Odontogenic fibroma

It is important that the differential diagnosis not be limited to these conditions but include others that may present in a similar fashion.

Although a definitive diagnosis of the lesion can only be based on a histologic examination, a reasonably accurate clinical diagnosis can be determined if the following conditions exist:

1. A periapical lesion involved with one or more nonvital teeth
2. A lesion greater than 200 mm^2 in size
3. A lesion seen radiographically as a circumscribed, well-defined radiolucent area, bounded by a thin radiopaque line
4. A lesion that produces a straw-colored fluid upon aspiration or that drains through an accessed root canal system

Treatment options to manage large cystic lesions range from nonsurgical root canal therapy to apical surgery to extraction.

An alternative plan of treatment and a more conservative approach is a *decompression* procedure. This procedure allows for continuous drainage, which removes those conditions that favor cyst expansion.

Surgical technique notes

Anesthesia

Although block anesthesia is ideal for this procedure, a topical anesthetic can be placed over the center of the surgical site, followed by a localized subcutaneous infiltration; this combination produces more than an adequate level of anesthesia.

Aspiration

An aspirant of a straw-colored fluid confirms the provisional diagnosis of a large cystic lesion. It may be straw colored, cloudy, or a combination of a serosanguinous purulent mixture. Repeated aspirations of blood or failure to withdraw any fluid indicate that the provisional diagnosis should be reevaluated. The absence of any aspirant may indicate a fibrous or any solid cellular lesion. Large radiolucent lesions should never be entered before they are aspirated.

Decompression tube fabrication

The decompression tube maintains drainage and facilitates repeated irrigation. Fabrication consists of a section of tubing from a standard intravenous setup. This type of tubing is used because it is noncollapsible, is sufficient in diameter to prevent clogging, and is readily available. It also facilitates insertion and removal and can be adjusted and fashioned for patient comfort. Various lengths of the tubing are precut. A beveled terminal insertable end is fabricated by sectioning one end of the tube at a 45-degree angle. On the opposite end of the tube, an external button is formed by briefly applying the heated end of a spatula. The button can be angled, depending on the anatomic contours. The tubing is then sterilized and ready for placement.

Incision

An incision is made with a no. 11 blade directed into the center of the lesion. A vertical incision is made through the periosteum to bone and usually penetrates into the defect. On occasion the underlying bone may require perforation with a round bur before the tube can be placed. Initial drainage usually occurs at this time.

Decompression tube insertion

The beveled end of the tube (sufficient in length) is inserted using a slight rotary motion. It is directed into the depth of the lesion until resistance is met at the posterior wall of the defect. Adjustment is made until the button is flush with the external tissue; this can be determined by removing the tube and adjusting the length at the beveled end and reinserting it until the button is flush. On occasion a suture may be required, either above or below the tube on the vertical incision line, to ensure close adaptation of the tissue.

Irrigation

The patient is instructed on the proper irrigation technique. A 10-mL disposable *Luer-Lok* syringe with an irrigating needle is prescribed for the patient along with a supply of sterile saline. The patient should irrigate a minimum of three times daily using the entire contents of a 10-mL syringe. The patient is monitored on a weekly basis until there is no additional evidence of debris or cystic contents flushed from the lesion. This course of treatment normally lasts 2 to 4 weeks. During this period of observation the tube can be easily removed by the clinician for inspection and cleansed, if required, then reinserted without difficulty. The patient is instructed in standard oral hygiene techniques and reappointed.

Endodontic therapy

Ideally, endodontic therapy should be completed after tube placement. This will ensure a dry canal prior to obturation and prevent the occurrence of posttreatment flare-up.

Tube removal

When drainage from the lesion ceases, the tube is removed. The remaining soft tissue defect should heal within a few days to a week.

Special considerations

Decompression procedures in the area of the maxillary first molars must be approached with caution. The anatomic position of the maxillary sinus and its radiographic superimposition over and in association with a large lesion can be misleading. Panographic and altered-angulation radiographs must be used in the evaluation and diagnosis. As long as the maxillary sinus can be identified and clearly separated from the periapical lesion, the chances of a perforation into the sinus and the creation of an oral-antral fistula can be avoided.

Followup

The patient is placed on 3-month followup observation and is checked radiographically for signs of osseous repair. The rate of healing depends on many factors and will vary from individual to individual. Failure of the lesion to resolve may necessitate surgical intervention and biopsy.

Preoperative Radiograph Examination

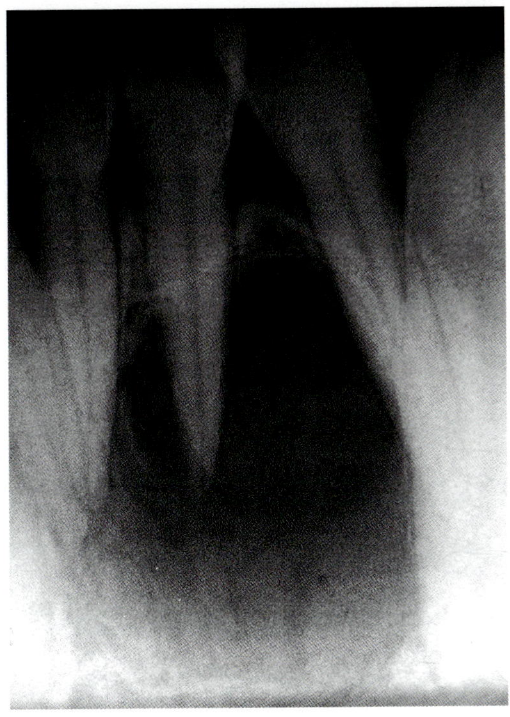

- Evaluate for:
  - radiolucent lesion associated with a nonvital tooth
  - a lesion 225 mm^2 in size and well defined
  - extension of the lesion, incorporating adjacent vital structures

Presurgical Soft Tissue Examination

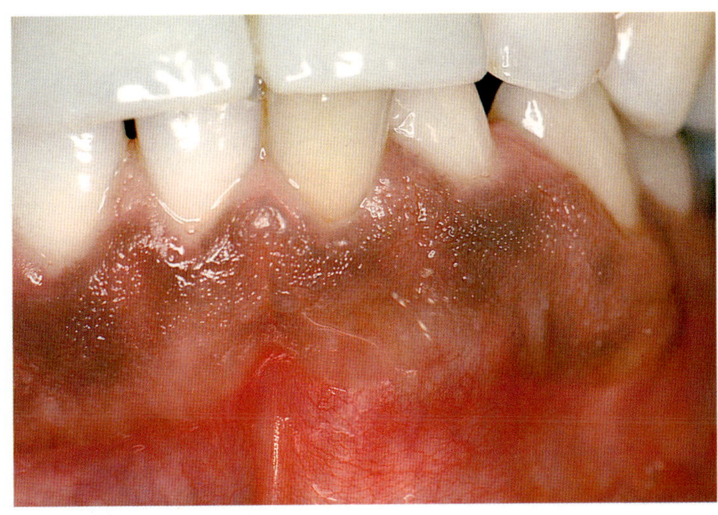

- Palpation reveals:
  - crepitation
  - pathologic fenestration
  - expansion of the lesion

Anesthesia

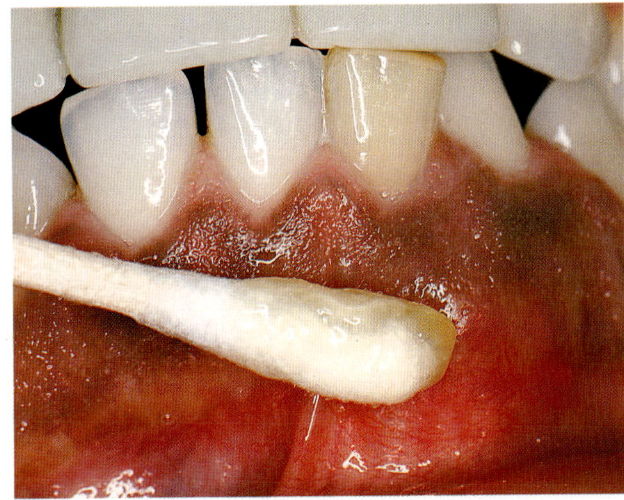

- Topical anesthesia.

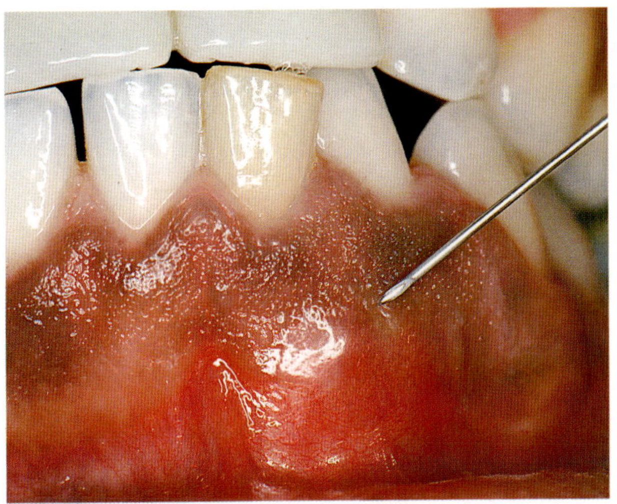

- Subcutaneous infiltration.

Aspiration of the Lesion

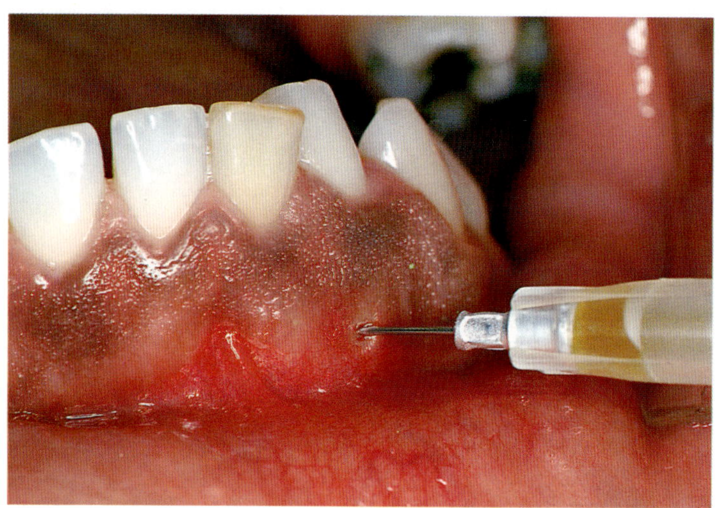

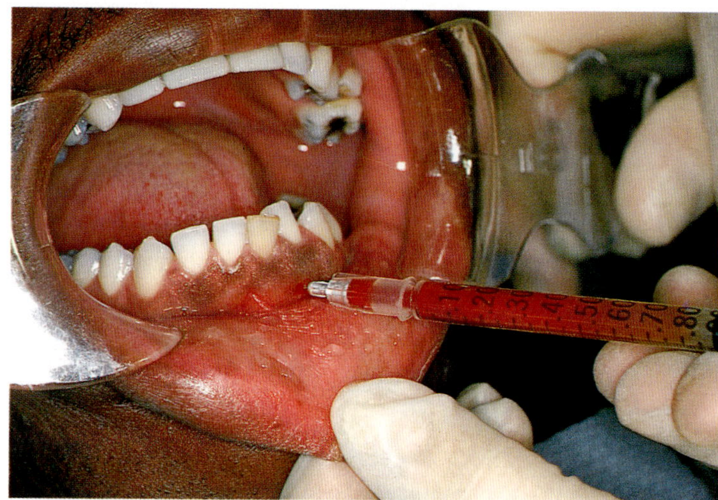

- Soft tissue and bony penetration.
- Slow, controlled aspiration of lesion contents.
- Aspirant consistent with provisional diagnosis.

Decompression Tube Fabrication

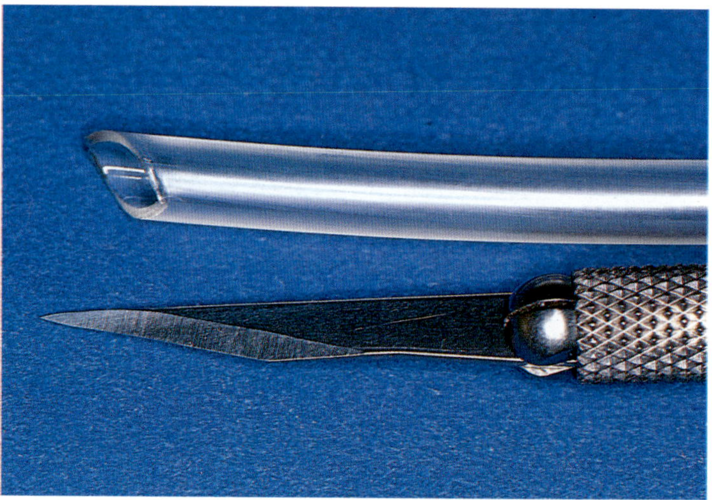

Beveled Terminal Insert

- Facilitates drainage.
- Enhances placement.

External Button Fabrication

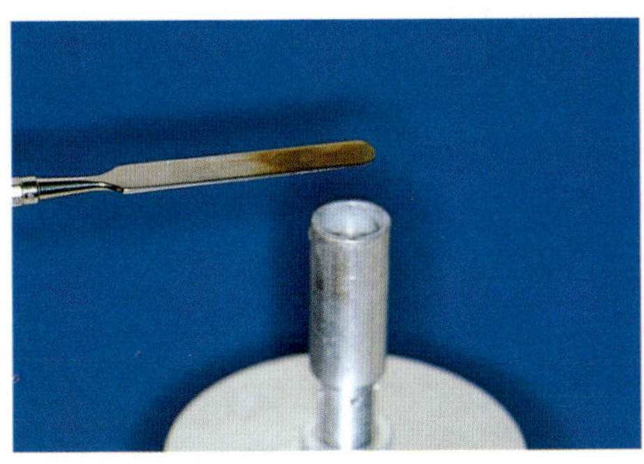

- Flat-ended spatula.
- Medium heat.

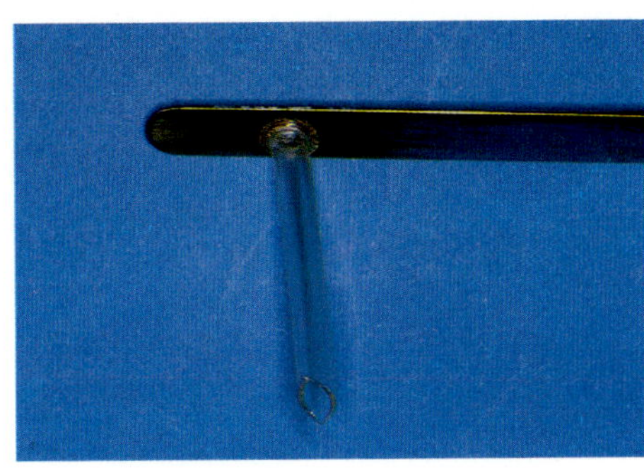

- Light compression against spatula, creating the button.

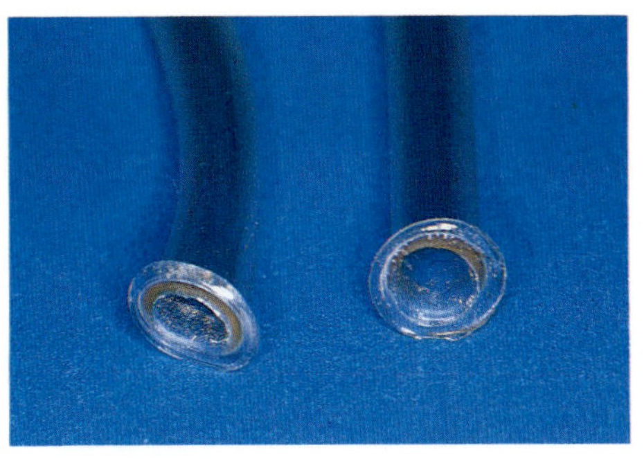

- Advantages:
  - prevents tube slippage
  - facilitates retention
- Angled depending on anatomic contours.

Blade Placement

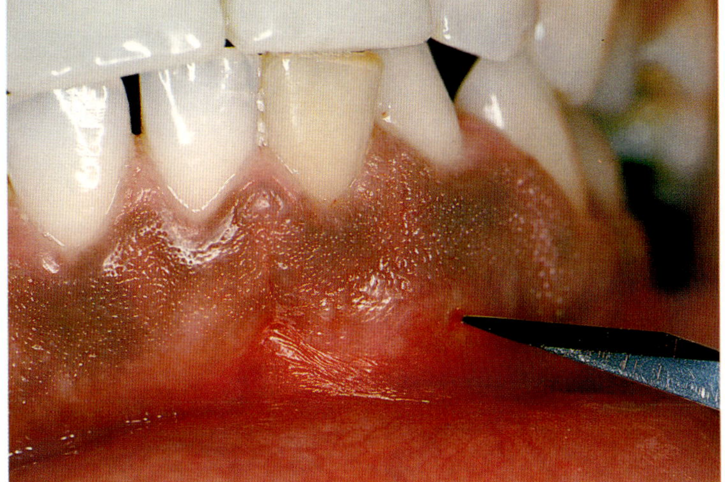

- Between root eminences.
- Direct toward center of lesion.

Incision

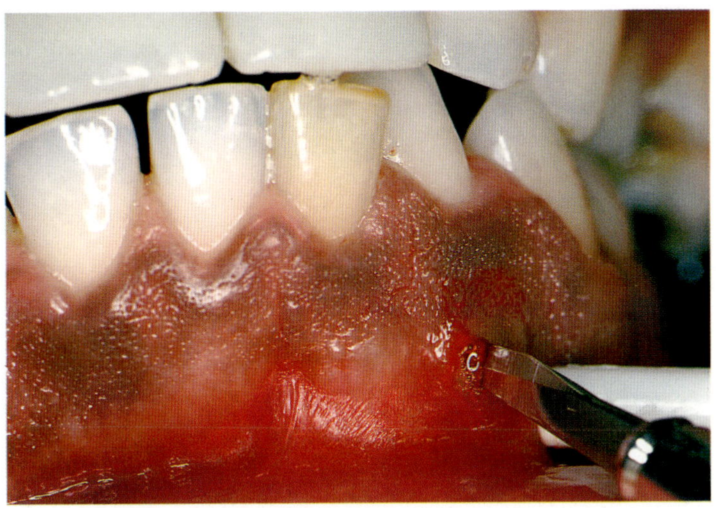

- Small, vertical incision to bone or into osseous fenestration.

Tube Insertion

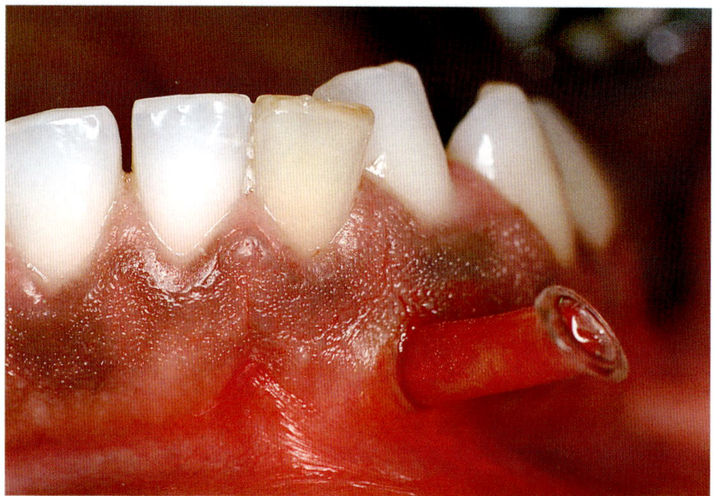

- Insert beveled end to depth of lesion.
- Measure excess tubing and adjust tube at beveled end.

Final Tube Placement

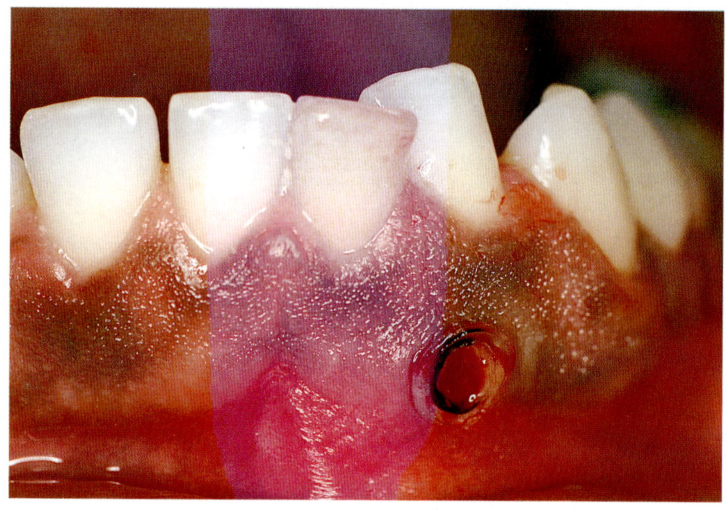

- Ensure functional drain is:
  - flush with mucosa
  - not overextended
  - patent

Irrigation

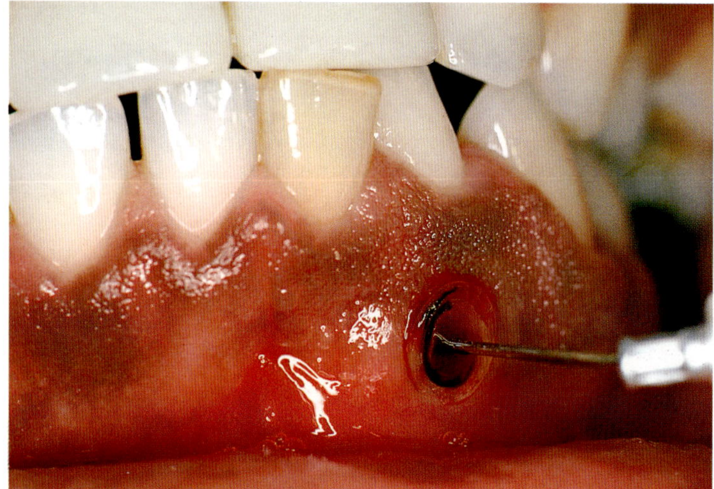

- Saline lavage.
- 10 mL three times daily.

Patient Instruction for Irrigation

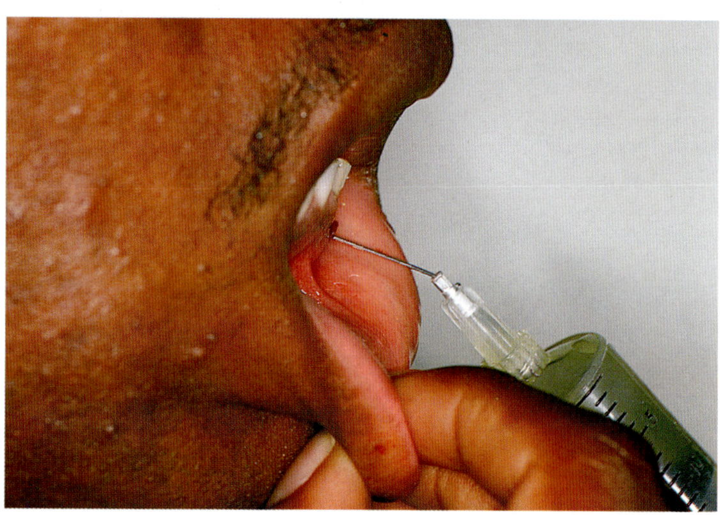

- A 10-mL syringe and sterile saline are prescribed for patient home care.
- Patient is instructed on proper irrigation and oral hygiene technique.

One-Day Followup

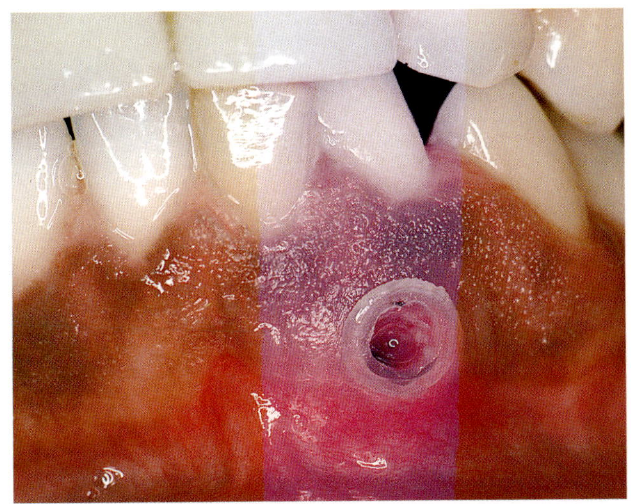

• Tube in place.

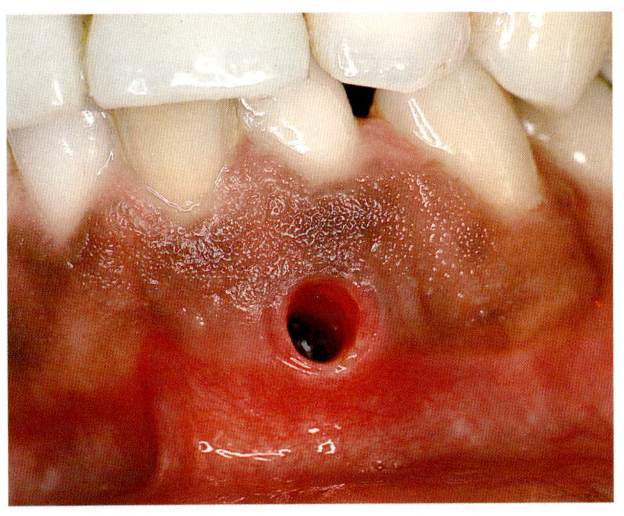

• Tubing removed showing epithelial collar and minimal inflammation.

One-Week Followup

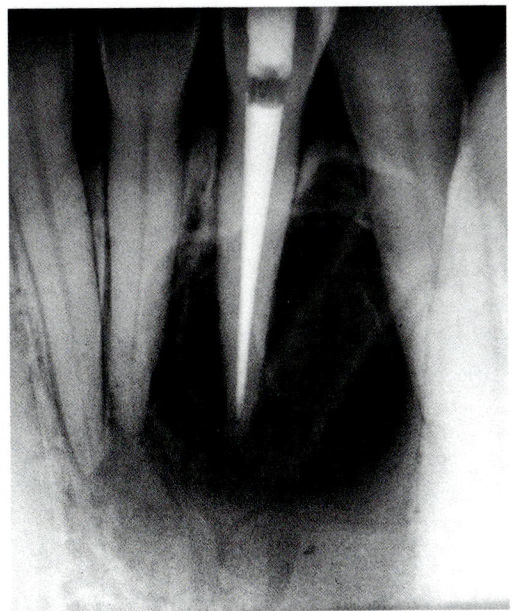

• Routine nonsurgical endodontics performed with tube in place.

Three-Month Followup

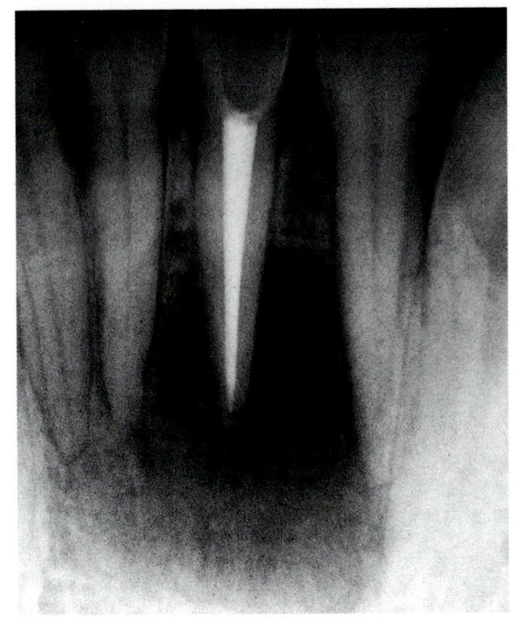

• Lesion decreasing in size.
• Displaced roots realigning.

Clinical Case of Healing Using the Decompression Technique (1-Year Followup)

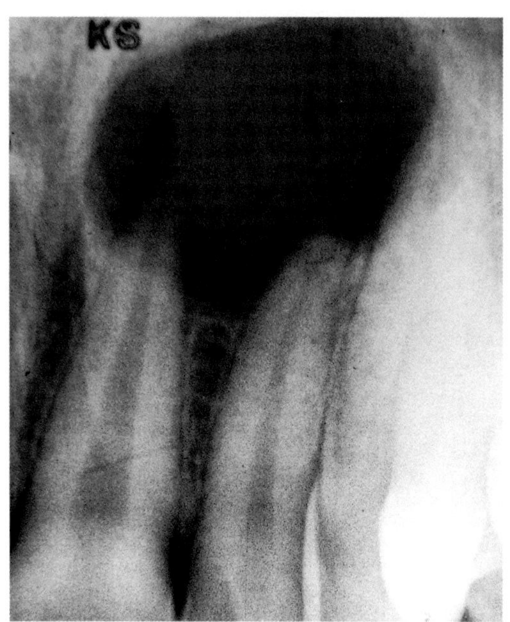

• Preoperative radiograph.

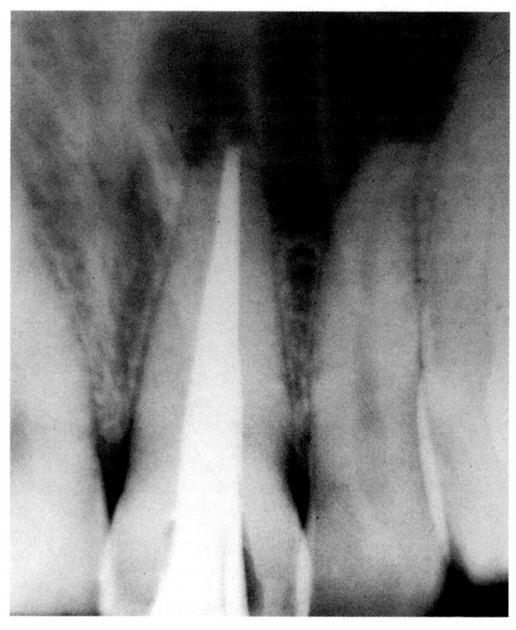

• Obturation with tube in place.

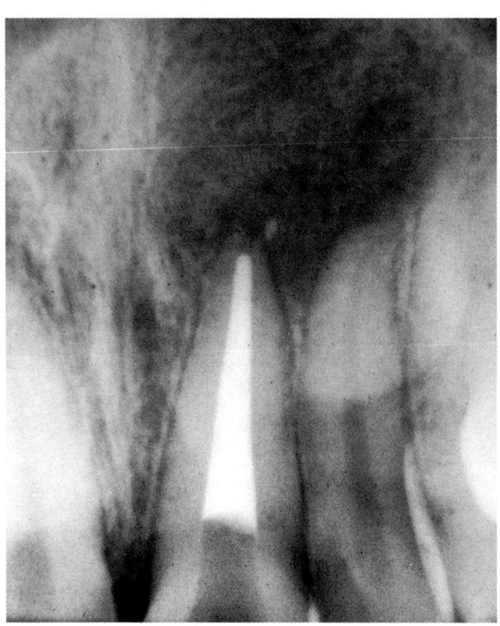

• One-year followup radiograph.

8 Maxillary Anterior Surgery

The majority of endodontic surgery is performed in the anterior maxilla. Anterior teeth are also the most frequently re-treated teeth. Often times, surgery is a part of this re-treatment, further complicating what is often referred to as a "routine procedure."

Significant anatomic structures encountered in the anterior maxilla are the floor of the nasal cavity, nasal spine, incisal and canine fossae, canine eminence, and incisal foramen. The cortical bone varies in thickness along the anterior maxilla, and it is very important to take this thickness variability into account.

The maxillary central incisor seems to present the least degree of surgical difficulty. The root is not excessively long, it is distant from the floor of the nasal cavity, and it has a moderate covering of cortical bone. These factors allow for easy access and provide the best visual field for apical surgery.

The lateral incisor has a smaller coronal dimension. The root is angled distally and is accompanied by a distopalatal inclination, which is curved more often than not. The root is usually housed deeper into the medullary bone, and access is frequently hampered by hemorrhage and a compromised visual field.

The maxillary canine has a longer root compared to its anterior analogs. The root has a prominent eminence that must be taken into account during flap design, repositioning, and suturing. The apex of the maxillary canine is located high upon the maxilla, where access and visibility are limited and cortical bone is thicker. Retraction may cause facial discoloration and swelling due to impingement on muscle attachments and tissue bulk, limiting vertical reflection. Retrograde amalgam placement must take into consideration the cross-sectional diameter of the root and the large oval canal. Suturing over the canine eminence stretches the thin ends of the flap, thus compromising the blood supply and predisposing the edges to tearing during suturing. For these reasons, avoid suturing over the canine eminence.

Surgical techniques notes

Flap design

A flap design should allow maximum visibility. When no prosthetic crowns are present, a full-thickness mucoperiosteal rectangular flap is recommended for maximum visibility. When prosthetic crowns are present, the Ochsenbein-Luebke flap should be considered as an alternative. Semilunar flaps are also popular, but they tend to limit visibility.

Incision

Make all incisions with a controlled, measured motion through mucosa to bone. Place vertical incisions not less than one tooth lateral to the tooth undergoing surgery and possibly more, depending on the degree of visibility and access required. Make incisions between, not on, prominent eminences. Place the horizontal component of the incision intrasulcularly, using the labial contours of the teeth as a guide. Use caution as the incision approaches the interproximal area where the papilla is carefully freed. In comparison to other areas of the mouth, the maxillary anterior region provides better than average visibility, a broad band of attached gingiva, and prominent labial contours, which act as guides for the intrasulcular and interproximal incisions.

Flap reflection

The marginal gingiva is firmly attached and can be difficult to reflect. Hold a quartered 2 x 2 gauze pack firmly over the tissue and direct reflection against it to prevent perforations and tissue tears. Buttressed and irregular bone contours can hamper reflection. In cases of long roots, impingement on the nasal spine and frenum attachments may compromise flap reflection.

Flap retraction

The retractor must always be placed perpendicular to bone to avoid impinging the periosteum and/or the flap. The flap should rest freely on the concave surface of the retractor so as not to crush or fold the papilla. The retractor should always rest firmly on the bone above the root apex and the pathologic defect.

Cortical bone exploration

Explore the surface of the cortical bone for a pathologic fenestration. If the bone is intact, probe it with an endodontic explorer to locate any area of reduced density that may be used to aid in root end localization.

Osseous access

Never begin initial bone removal at the estimated apex of the tooth. Use a presurgical radiograph to estimate the root length; this measurement can then be superimposed on the surgical site. Use the bony contour of the root in the apical third as a guide. Initial bone removal should expose the root surface, which is used as a guide to the apex. Once the apical third of the root is uncovered to the apex, enlarge the apical preparation, thus exposing the root apex.

Root end exposure

Identify and define the apical and lateral boundaries of the root. This step is basic to any type of apical surgery. If the root and apex cannot be defined, root resection should never be attempted. Periapical lesions should be enucleated and histologically examined.

Root resection

Resect the root at about a 45-degree angle to allow for root end visualization and subsequent root end preparation. Make the resection with a fissure bur in a straight handpiece with a clean continuous cut.

Root end inspection

Define the cut root end in its circumference using an endodontic explorer. Check the resection to ensure that the apical third of the root has been removed completely. The root canal in its cross-sectional diameter can now be visualized.

Root end preparation

Use a rotary instrument to prepare a Class I or slot preparation to receive the retrograde obturation material. Undercut the preparation to ensure retention. Then dry the apical preparation with the cut end of a paper point held in place by a cotton pliers.

Retrograde obturation

Establish hemorrhage control with either *Nu Gauze,* bone wax, *Gelfoam,* or *Surgicel.* The packing may be cut at different lengths and packed into the apical region. Dry the canal again with paper points. Obturate the apical preparation with the retrograde material of choice by means of the miniamalgam carrier or plastic instrument and condense it into place. The condensing instruments (pluggers) can be custom made from no. 23 explorers cut at different lengths.

During amalgam placement, never scrape or use a bur to remove the excess amalgam because the amalgam will become ingrained into the bone and then cannot easily be removed. Instead, irrigate copiously and use suction to remove the excess amalgam debris.

After placing the retrograde obturation material, irrigate the surgical site with saline, especially under the flap where debris tends to accumulate. Before final closure and suturing, always take a postoperative confirmation radiograph. Remove hemorrhage control packing at this time.

Final closure

Suture the flap to place using a single suspensory suture around the involved tooth. Then use standard interrupted sutures interproximally and along the vertical component, as needed. Reposition and apply gentle pressure to the flap during the entire suturing sequence to ensure continued adaptation and alignment.

Presurgical Radiographic Examination

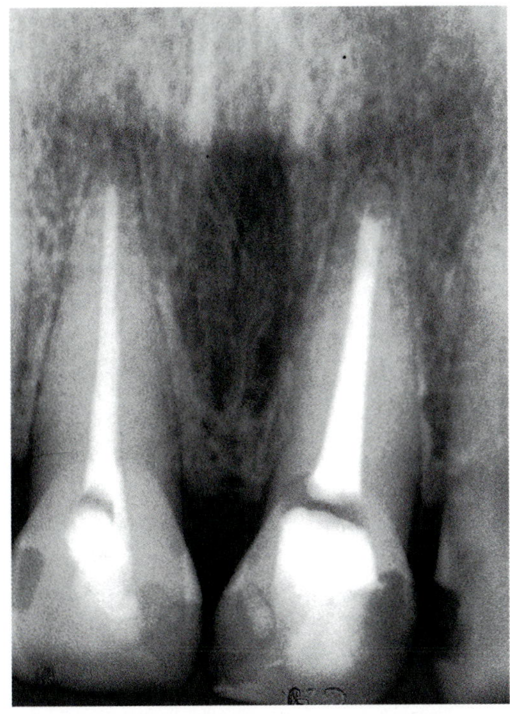

- Assess adequacy of root canal filling.
- Evaluate condition of adjacent teeth.
- Determine presence of apical pathology.
- Estimate length and anatomic position of surgically involved tooth.

Presurgical Soft Tissue Examination

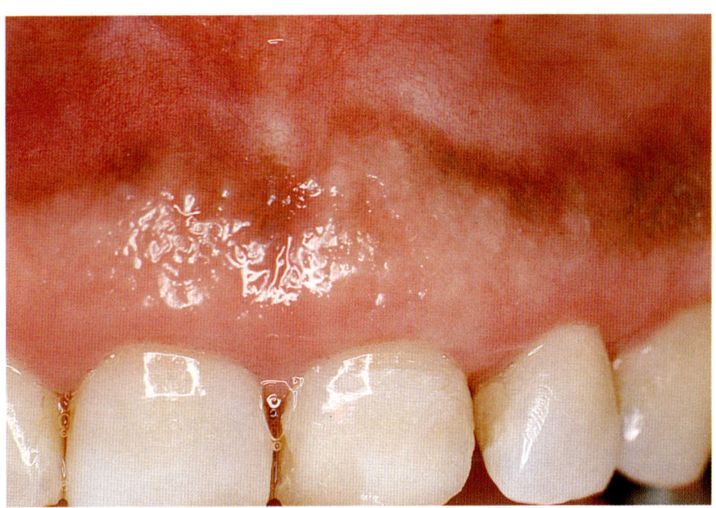

- Examination reveals:
  - broad band of attached gingiva
  - high muscle attachments
  - intact, noninflamed periodontium

Hard Tissue Anatomy

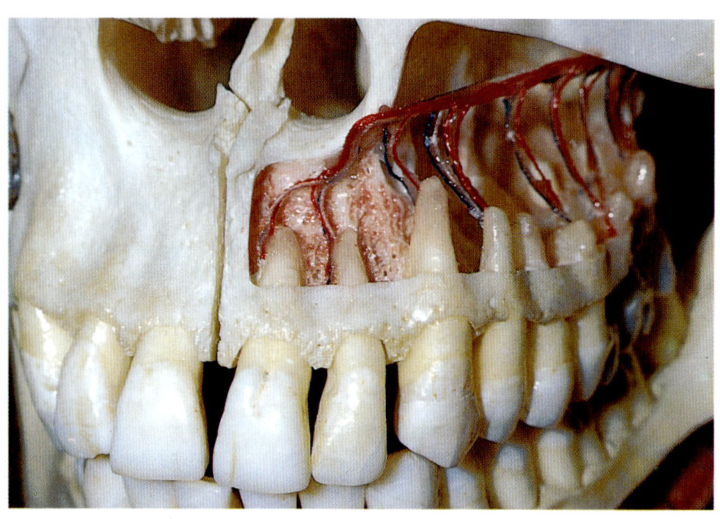

- Nasal cavity.
- Nasal spine.
- Neurovascular supply.
- Root length.

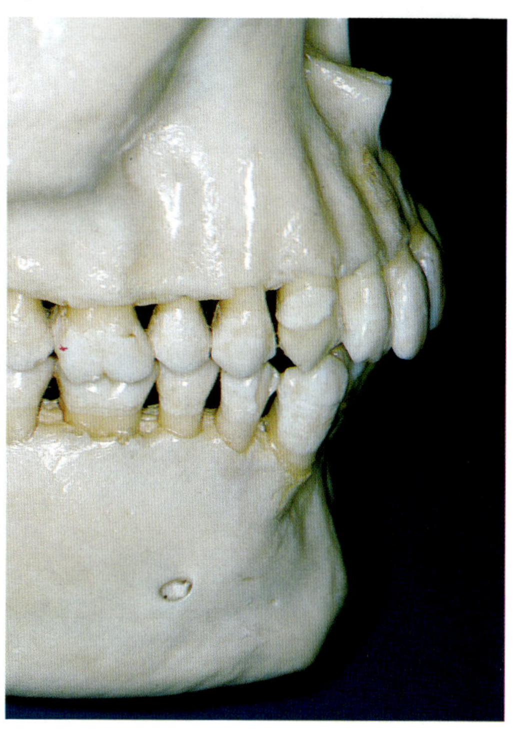

- Incisal and canine fossa.
- Canine eminence.
- Root inclination.
- Cortical bone thickness.

Position of Anterior Teeth in Bony Housing

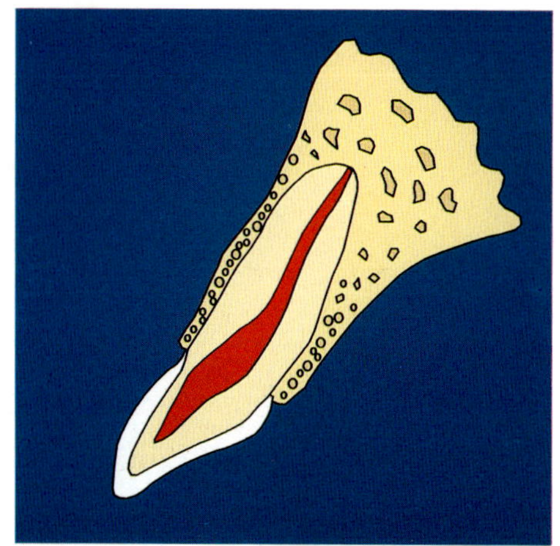

- Maxillary central incisor.

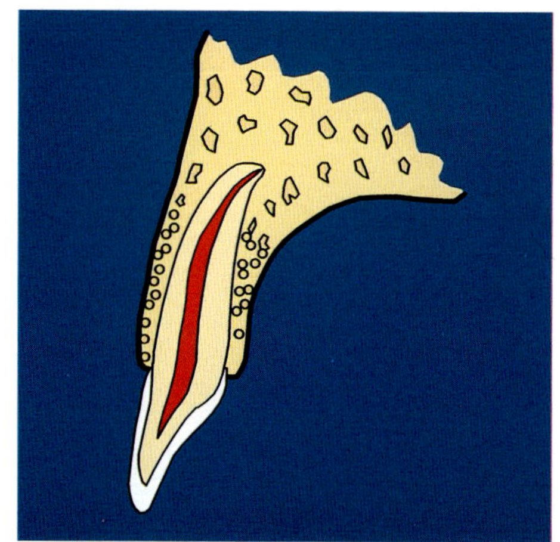

- Maxillary lateral incisor.

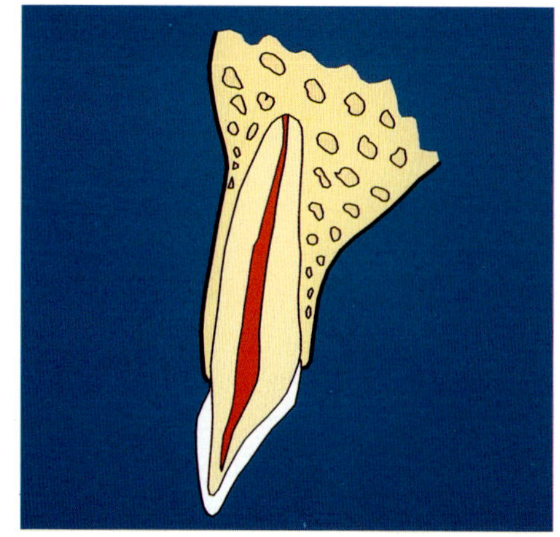

- Maxillary canine.

Rectangular Flap Design

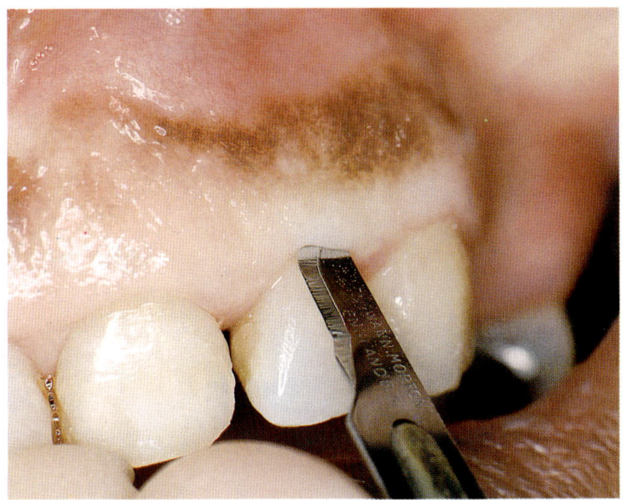

- Intrasulcular.
- Incise to level of crestal bone.

Vertical Incisions

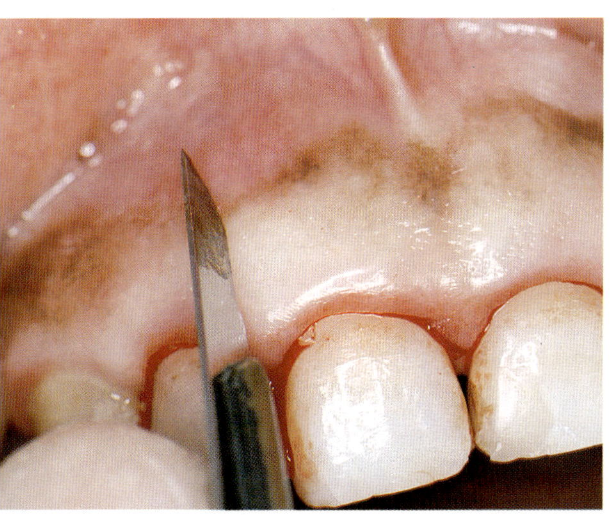

- Minimal extension into alveolar mucosa.
- Complete penetration of mucoperiosteum to bone.
- Place between root eminences.

Initial Flap Reflection

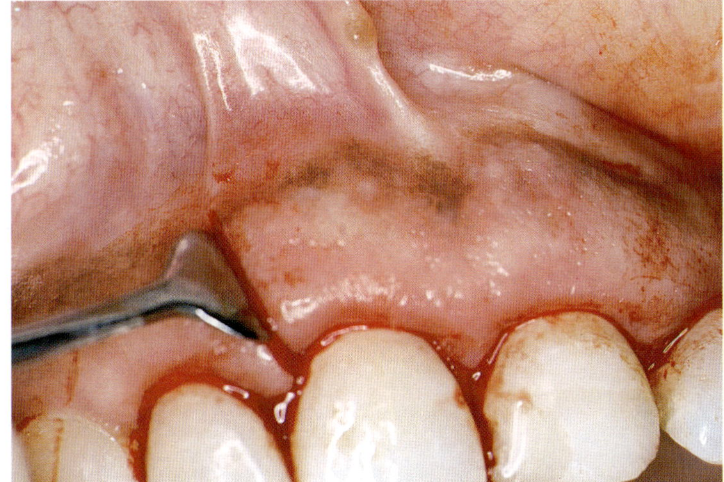

- Begin at midportion of vertical incision.
- Complete separation of periosteum from bone.
- Use undermining elevation, directed superiorly.

Flap Reflection

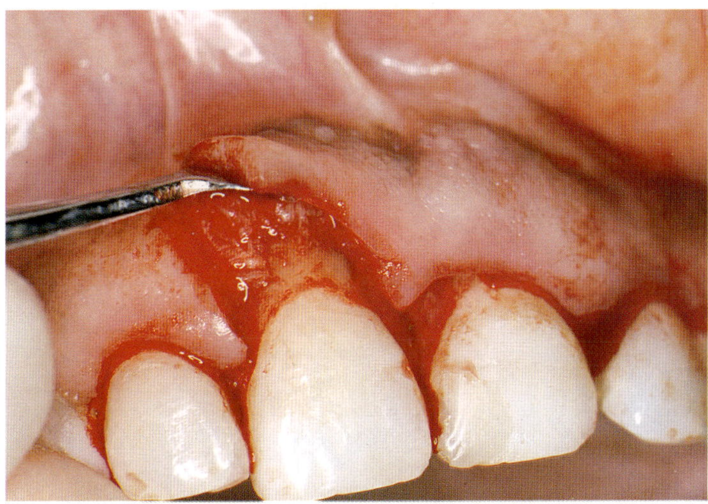

- Perform gentle and atraumatic reflection.
- Use care when reflecting over:
  - —irregular bone
  - —buttressed bone
  - —nasal spine

Flap Retraction

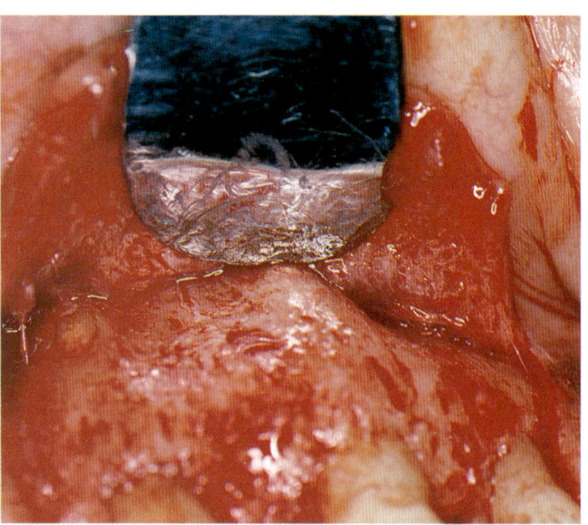

- Place the retractor perpendicular to bone.
- Place retractor firmly onto bone.
- Avoid soft tissue impingement.

Exploration of Cortical Bone

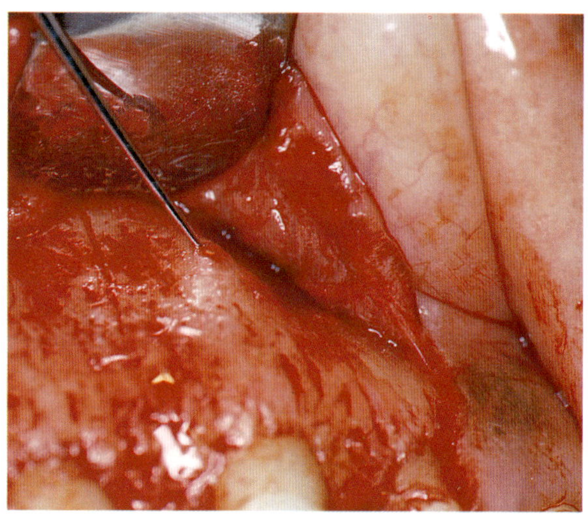

- Cortical bone determination:
  - intact
  - pathologic fenestration
  - physiologic fenestration

Decortication of Overlying Bone

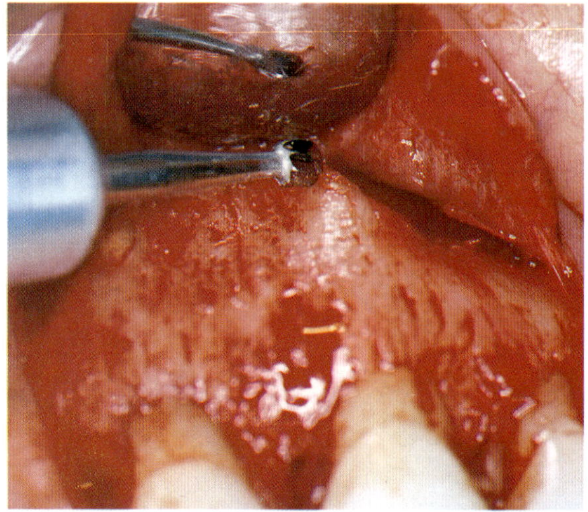

- Measure endometrically before bone removal.
- Use root contours as a guide for initial bone removal.
- Make osseous access to apical third.
- Identify root surface and remove bone apically.

Root End Exposure

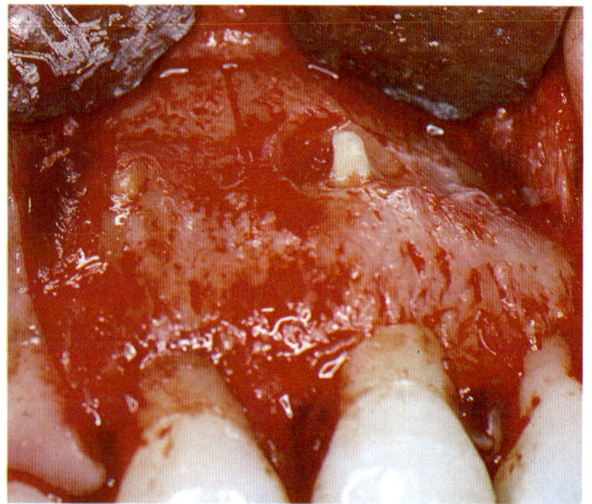

- Define lateral and apical limits of the root apex.
- Visualize apical lesion (if present).
- Submit lesion for histologic exam.

Root Resection

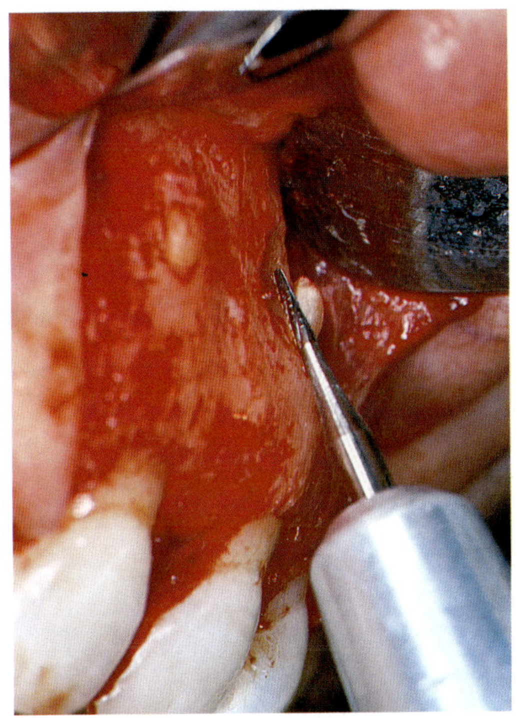

- Never resect a poorly defined root that is difficult to see.
- Place bevel so as to maximize visualization of root end.
- Resect in one complete plane using a fissure bur.

Root End Inspection

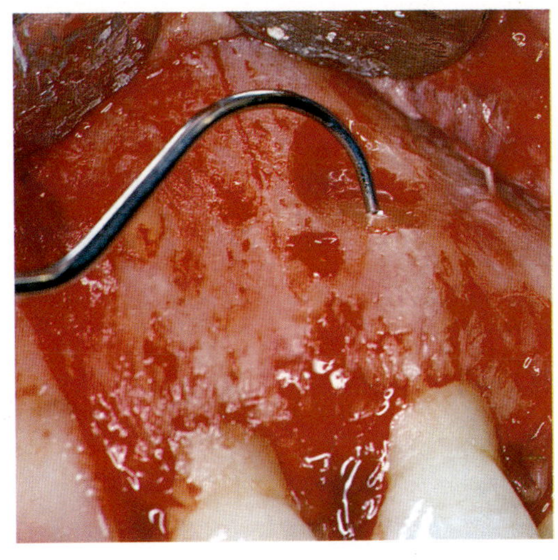

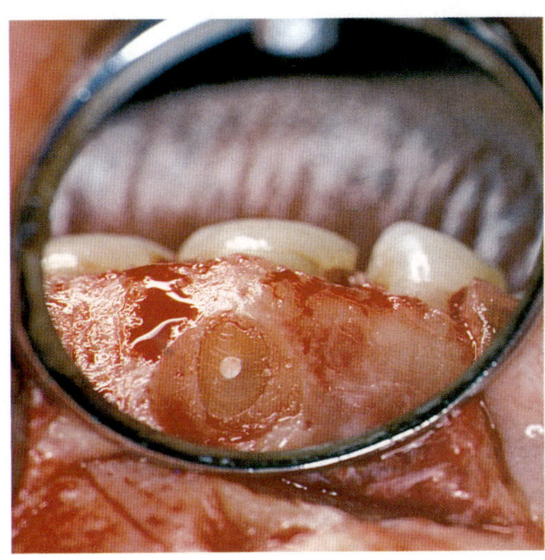

- Visualize lateral and posterior boundaries of the periodontium surrounding the root.
- Inspect for fractures, cracks, perforations, additional canals, and anatomic anomalies.
- Inspect existing obturation (when present).

Resected Roots of Maxillary Anterior Teeth

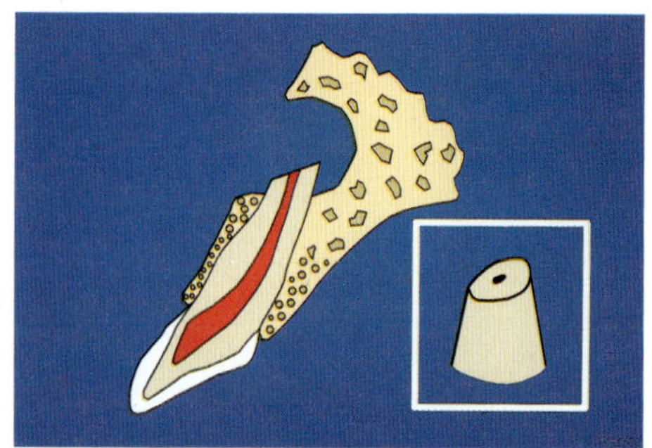

• Maxillary central incisor.

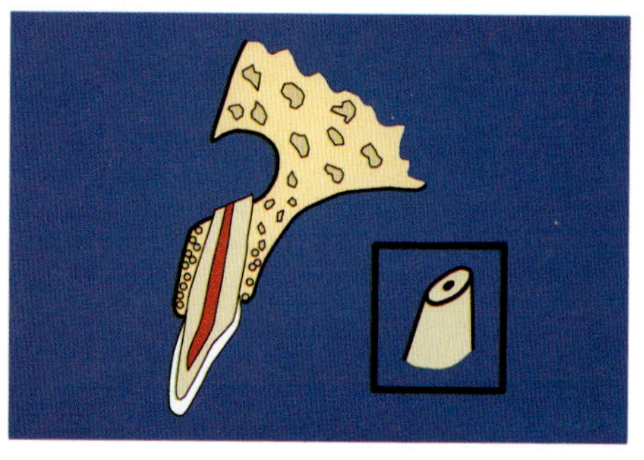

• Maxillary lateral incisor.

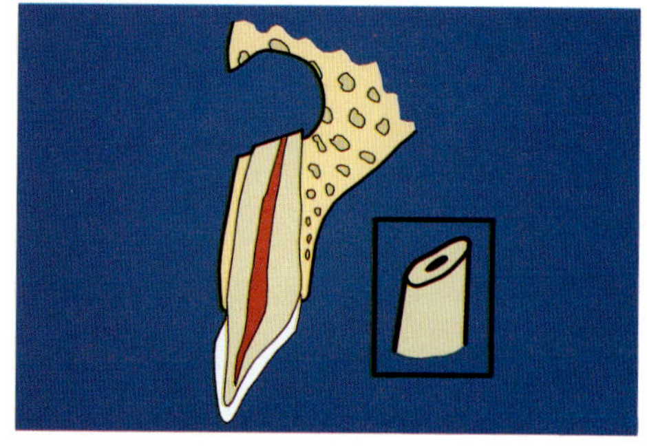

• Maxillary canine.

Apical Preparation

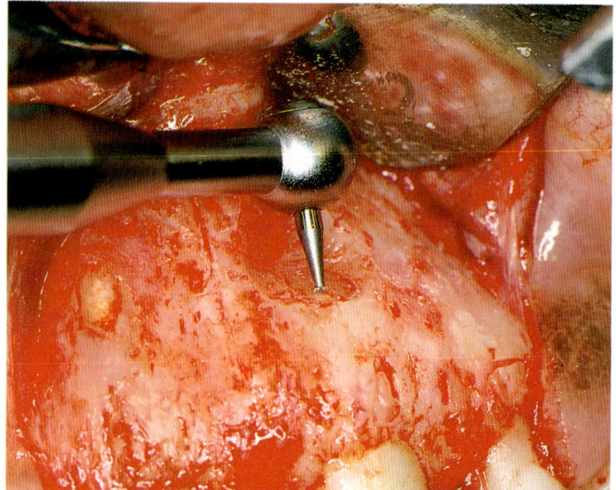

- Use microhead handpiece in restricted surgical site.
- Perform Class I preparation.
- Make preparation within canal, in line with long axis of root, to prevent perforation.
- Prepare mechanical undercut.

Drying the Apical Preparation

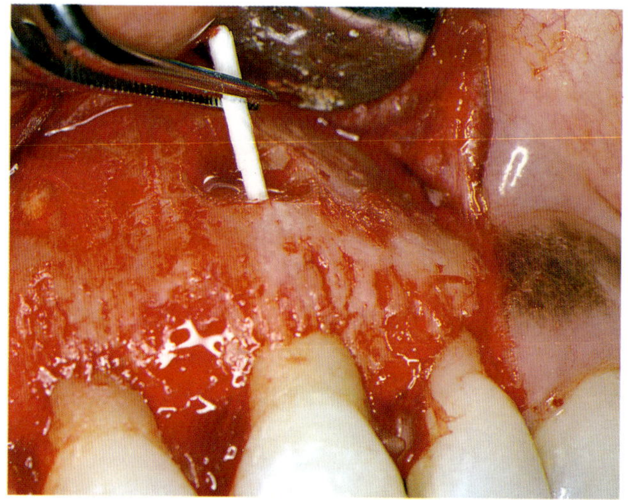

- Apical saline lavage.
- Maintain hemorrhage control to prevent contamination, using:
  — *Nu Gauze*
  — bone wax
  — *Gelfoam*
  — *Surgicel*
- Dry apical preparation with cut ends of paper points.

Amalgam Placement

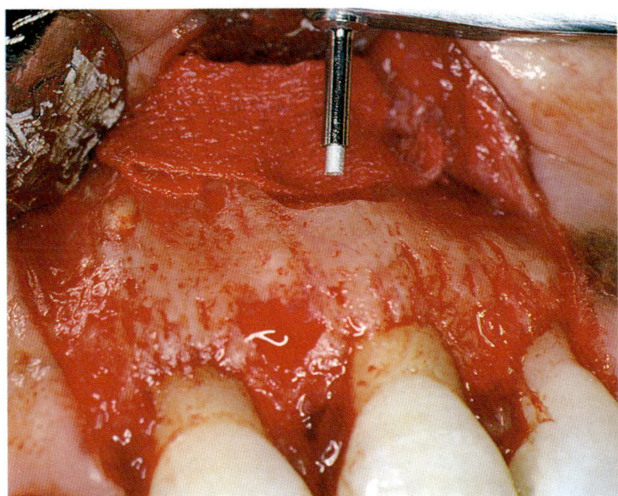

- Select retrograde material of choice:
  - amalgam
  - *IRM* (Intermediate Restorative Material)
  - gutta-percha (cold burnished)
- Use miniamalgam carrier.

Amalgam Condensation

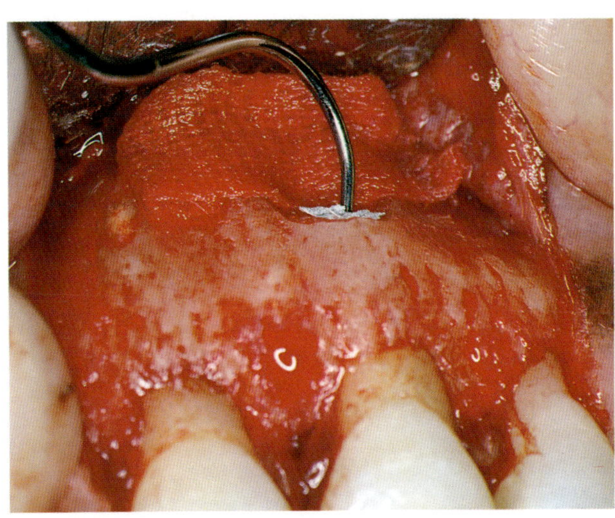

- Use modified explorer-condensers.
- Vertically compact amalgam.
- Remove excess amalgam by saline lavage and suction.

Completed Retrograde Obturation

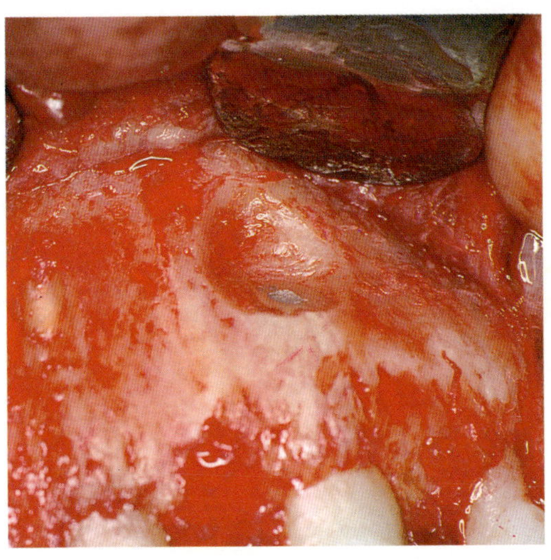

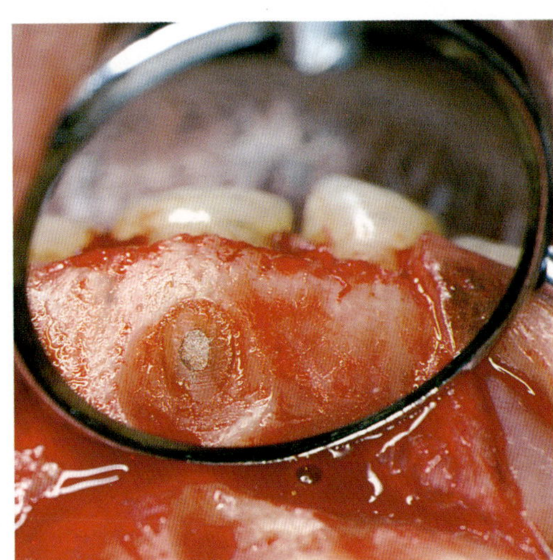

- Irrigate apical site and beneath flap.
- Clinically inspect retrograde obturation.
- Ensure absence of amalgam fragments and bone debris.
- Remove apical packing before repositioning the flap.

Radiographic Confirmation

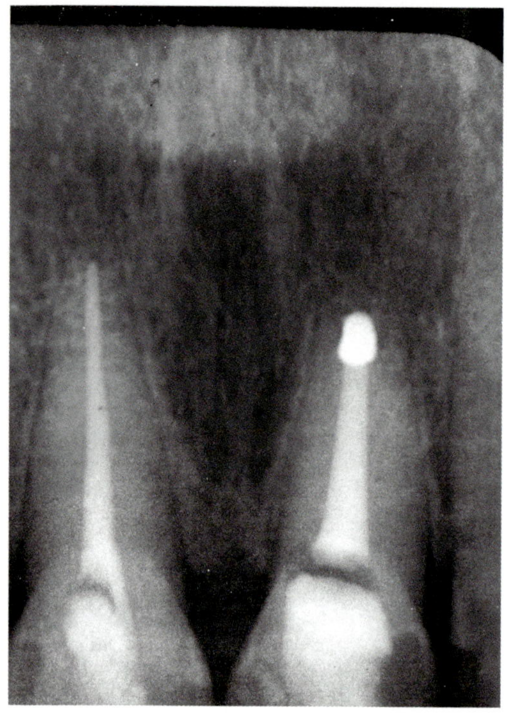

- Take radiograph before closure.
- Inspect for amalgam debris, complete resection, and position of retrograde filling.

Final Closure

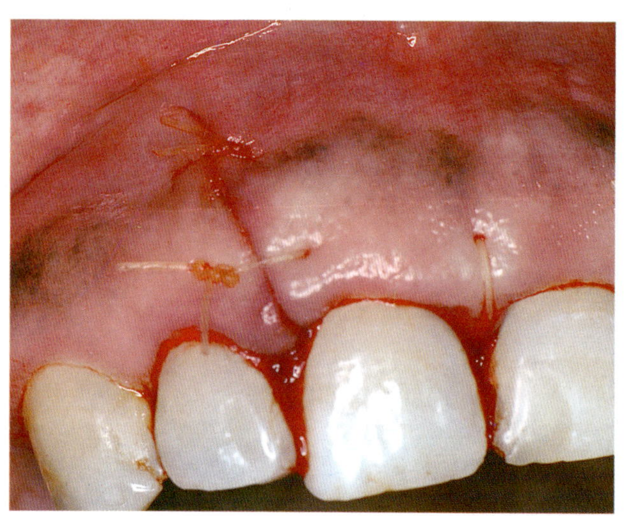

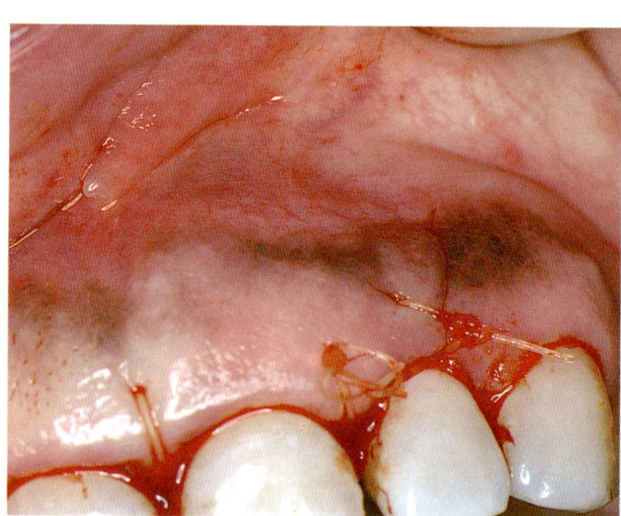

- Place single suspensory suture around surgically involved tooth.
- Place interrupted sutures interproximally and along vertical incisions as needed.

One Week Postsurgery

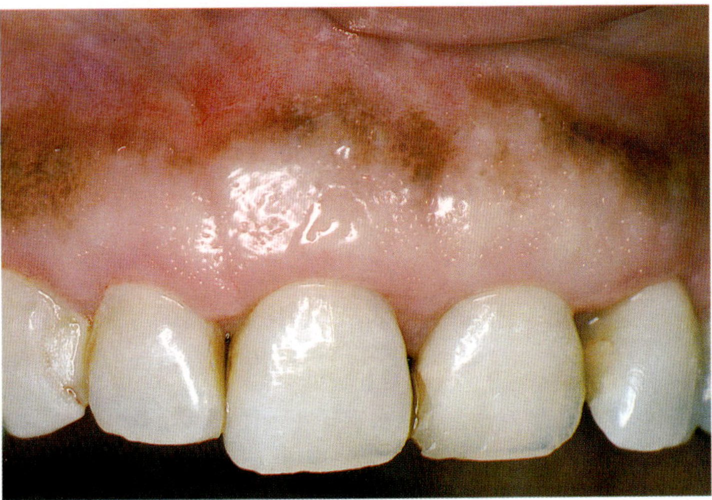

- Monitor soft tissue healing.
- Reinforce oral hygiene.

9 Mandibular Anterior Surgery

Surgical endodontic procedures performed in the anterior portion of the mandible present several difficulties not seen elsewhere in the oral cavity. Anatomic structures associated with the anterior portion of the mandible hamper an unobstructed access to the surgical site, contrary to what you might expect. Noteworthy structures are: the mental foramen, mental protuberance, mental tubercle, and root length with its lingual inclination. Additional considerations include prominent nutrient canals, cortical bone that thickens inferiorly toward the symphysis, buttressed bone along the alveolar crest, and muscle attachments.

The mandibular incisors can be considered one grouping for discussion purposes. The labial coronal inclination is an indicator that the roots have a distinctive lingual inclination that can compromise visibility. Although root length is not a major problem, root proximity is. Unfortunately, it is possible to resect the wrong root or to inflict bur damage to adjacent roots because of such proximity. Nutrient canals, when perforated or entered, can bleed into the surgical site, thus obstructing visibility and compromising access.

The mandibular canine presents with a long root, a prominent eminence, and usually thick cortical bone inferiorly. With this in mind, vertical incisions on the eminence should be avoided and the flap should be extended an additional tooth distally, if necessary. Reflection in this area can be made difficult by muscle attachments.

Mandibular anterior teeth, including canines, frequently have multiple canals. Differential diagnosis should always be made using angulation radiographs along with straight-on views; this will ensure indentification of a multiple canal system and is critical in retreatment cases to ensure that the second canal has been obturated before surgery. Apical resection and retrograde obturation is not a substitute for a three-dimensional root canal obturation. Mandibular anterior teeth with prosthetic crowns and posts should be evaluated for vertical root fractures and perforation; this must always be considered and the patient forewarned.

Surgical technique notes

Flap design

Either triangular or rectangular flaps are commonly used in this region. The shorter roots of the mandibular anterior teeth (especially the central and lateral incisors) make the triangular flap feasible. However, the triangular flap can limit visibility if it is not large enough. Flap design can be a problem especially in patients who have prosthetic crowns and/or pontics. The Ochsenbein-Luebke flap can be attempted only if there is a sufficient band of attached gingiva. Advise patients with prosthetic crowns that in spite of sound surgical techniques, recession may occur.

Incision

Place vertical incisions one or two teeth on either side of the tooth in question. Check the level of the muscle attachments before making an incision. High attachments may dictate wider flaps and incisions that avoid penetrating muscle. This will reduce swelling, pain, and bleeding postoperatively. It is not uncommon to have pronounced bony ridges along the alveolar crest as well as buttressed bone. Follow the labial contours of the teeth for the intrasulcular incision and use the mini-blade; these will ensure a free release of the marginal gingiva. However, exercise care when encountering the bony contours to avoid irregular incisions that do not adequately free the marginal or interproximal gingiva.

Flap reflection

Because the tissue on the anterior mandible is taut, reflect the flap with caution. Firmly hold a 2 × 2 quartered gauze on the tissue. Direct reflection with a no. 4 Molt curet against the gauze pack, which acts as a backstop and cushion, preventing tears and perforations. Muscle attachments may be encountered inferiorly and laterally. The concavity of the symphysis may impede a clean mucoperiosteal reflection. Use a sharp no. 4 Molt curet to facilitate a complete mucoperiosteal reflection.

Flap retraction

Place the retractor perpendicular to bone to avoid impinging the periosteum and soft tissue. Allow the flap to rest freely on the concave surface of the retractor.

Cortical bone exploration

Because the cortical bone is thin, the pathologic defects are usually more prominent and easily observed. Exploration of the cortical plate with an endodontic explorer may be required to localize the pathologic defect.

Osseous access

If a pathologic fenestration is present, it can be enlarged with a round bur of suitable size, isolating the apex. If a defect is not present, use the rule of thirds and utilize the apical third of the root as a guide to the apex.

Root end exposure

After the apex has been visualized and isolated, remove the apical lesion, if present. Submit the specimen for histologic examination.

Root resection

If apical access and visibility are inadequate, do not attempt to resect the root. The lingual inclination makes this step difficult if the root is not clearly defined and isolated. Make the cut at a 45-degree angle. Ensure the resected root is the one in question and avoid injury to adjacent teeth in close proximity.

Root inspection

The cross-sectional diameter of the mandibular anterior roots is elongated and oval. If the initial cut is not angled enough, any secondary canal may be overlooked.

Root end preparation

Because the cross-sectional diameter of the root of mandibular anterior teeth is small, apical preparation to receive a retrograde material can be difficult. A sufficient section of the root end must be resected at a reasonable level in order to present a cross-sectional surface sufficient enough to prepare a Class I retention form. If a slot preparation is considered, exercise care because of the narrow and elongated anatomy of the cut root. The lingual inclination complicates the approach to the preparation. The microhead handpiece is very useful within this confined area.

Retrograde obturation

Hemorrhage may be a problem in this area due to the presence of nutrient canals and the medullary bone in the region. Hemostasis can be established with *Nu Gauze,* bone wax, *Gelfoam,* or *Surgicel;* when these are packed carefully into the surgical site they create a pressure barrier sufficient to control bleeding. Seal the apex with the retrograde material of choice. Because of the lingual inclination of the roots, there is a greater chance for amalgam debris to be displaced into the bony defect. Because the bone is very medullar, the amalgam particles have a greater chance of being ingrained. A simple saline lavage and suction, rather than mechanical removal, will clear the debris with minimal difficulty. The hemorrhage-control packing can now be removed. Before final closure, take a postoperative radiograph.

Final closure

Repositioning the tissue and suturing take more time than you might expect. The bulk of the lower lip, a restricted surgical site, and the thinness of the tissue all complicate the procedure. Use a single suspensory suture around the involved tooth, followed by single interrupted sutures interproximally and vertically, as needed. The suturing sequence is the same as used in the maxillary anterior region.

Presurgical Radiographic Examination

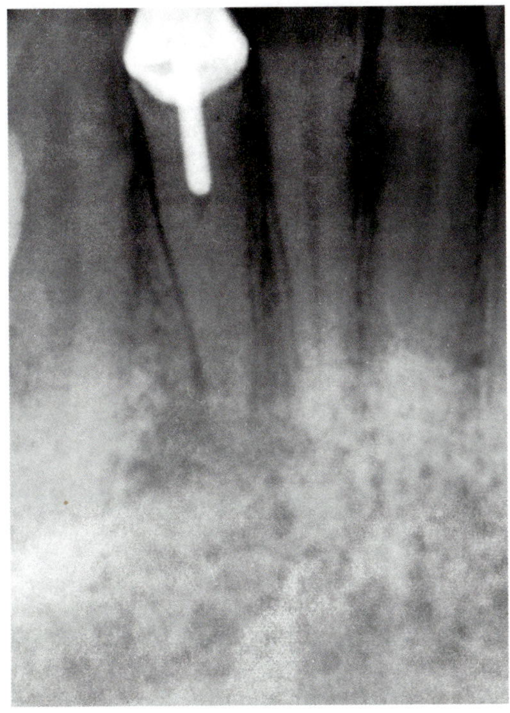

- Evaluate for:
  - root length and position
  - prosthetic crown with post
  - obstructed canal
  - periapical radiolucency

Presurgical Soft Tissue Examination

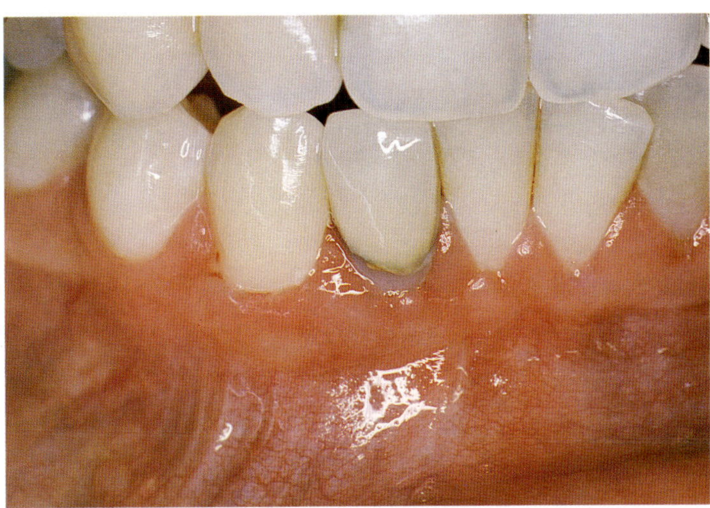

- Evaluate for:
  - muscle attachments
  - attached gingiva
  - gingival recession

Anatomic Landmarks

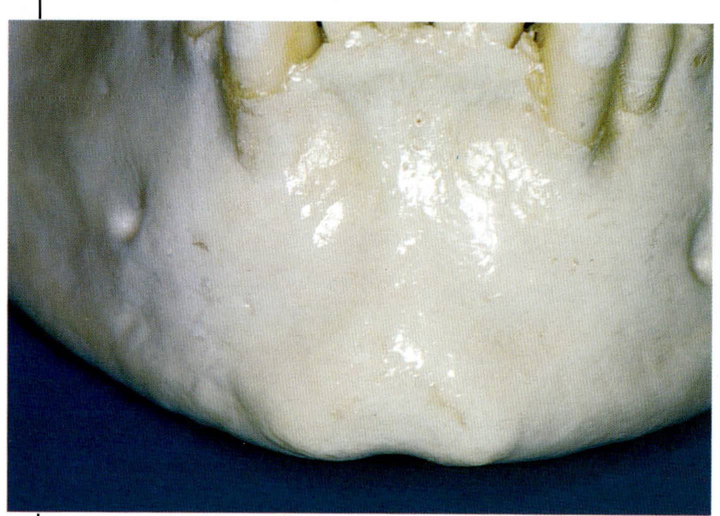

- Mental protuberance.
- Mental tubercles.
- Buttress bone.
- Mental foramen.
- Canine eminences.
- Thickness of cortical bone.

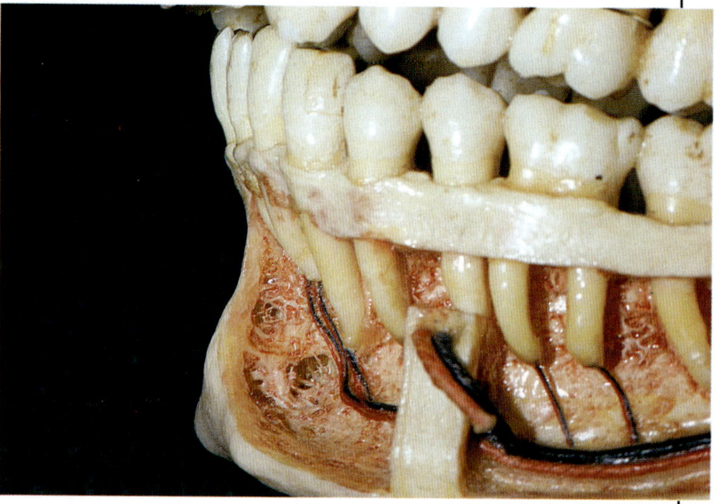

- Root length.
- Buccal lingual inclination.
- Position of apex.

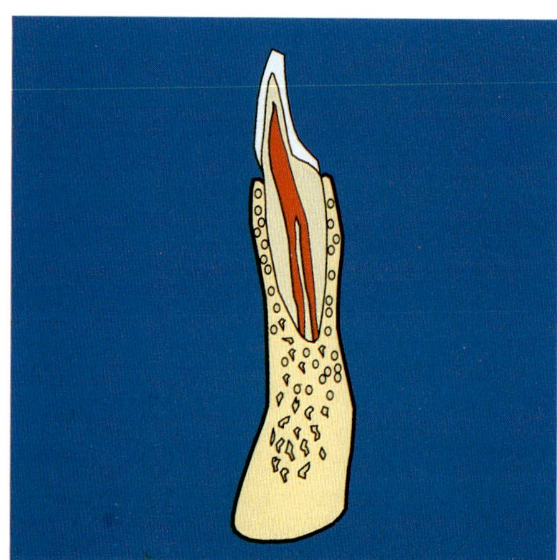

- Position of mandibular incisor within bony housing.

Flap Design

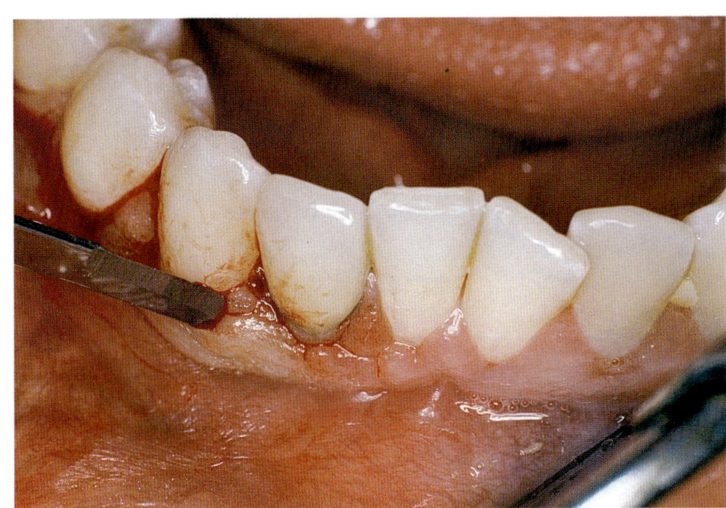

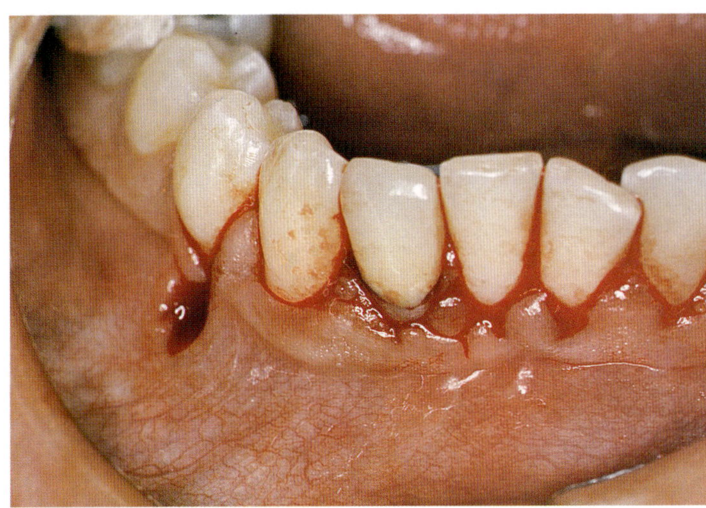

- Horizontal incision:
  - intrasulcular
  - use miniblade
- Vertical incision(s):
  - triangular flap
  - rectangular flap

Flap Reflection

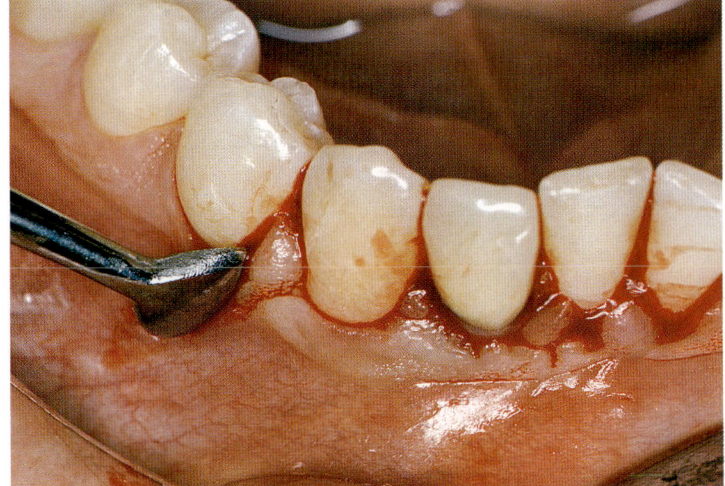

- Use a No. 4 Molt curet.
- Mid portion — vertical incision.
- Undermining elevation.

Flap Retraction

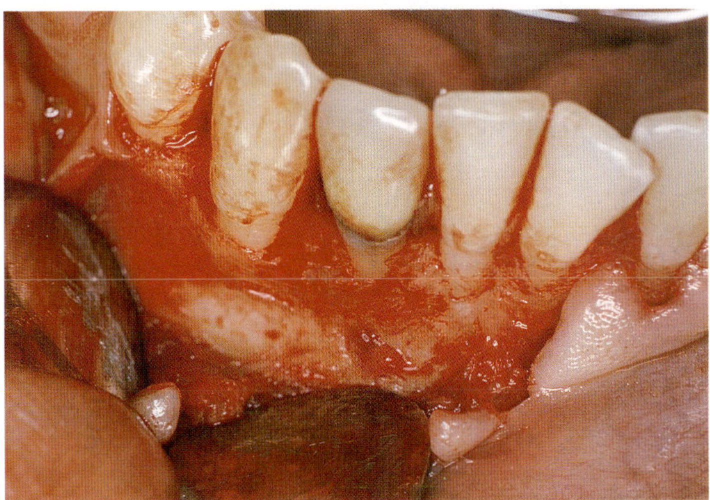

- Cortical bone visualization:
  - intact
  - dehiscence
  - pathologic fenestration
- Retractor placement:
  - perpendicular to bone
  - free of soft tissue impingement

Cortical Bone Removal

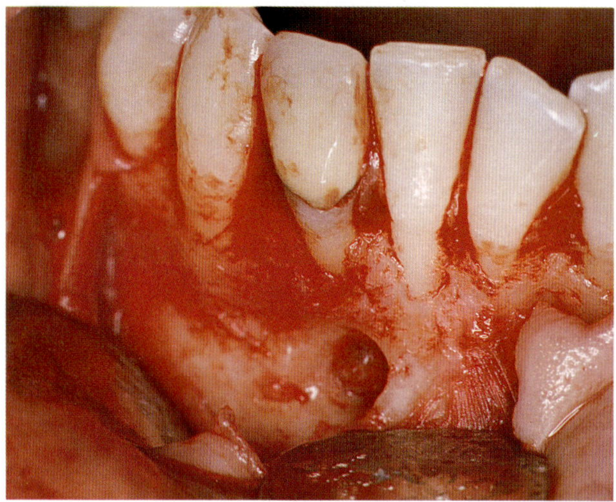

- Examine approximate root length.
- Use endometrics to approximate root length.
- Use root contour to locate apical third.

Root End Exposure

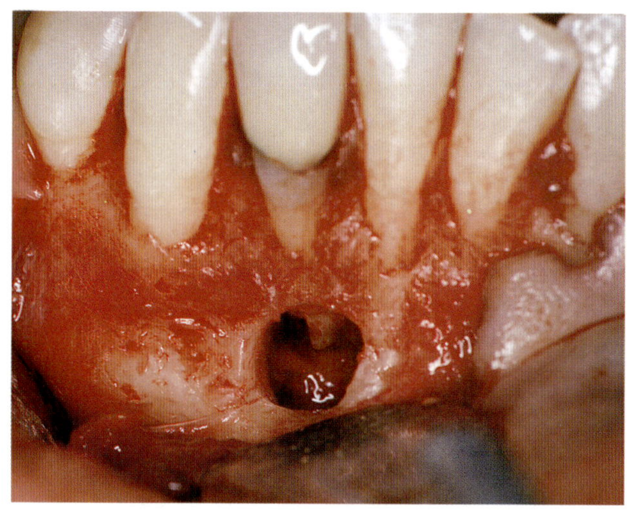

- Define root boundaries.
- Remove lesion and perform biopsy.
- Visualize apex.

Root Resection

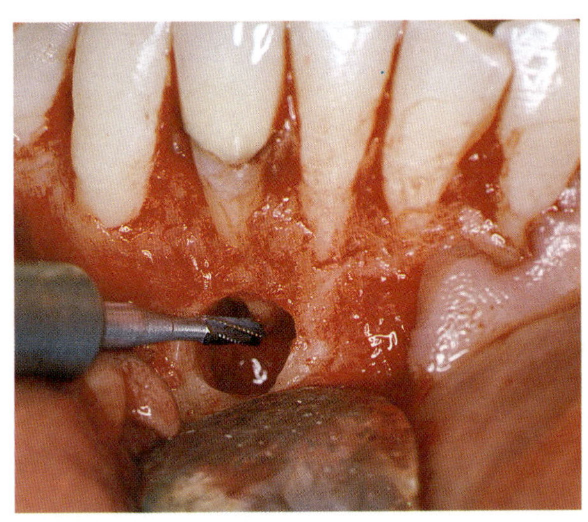

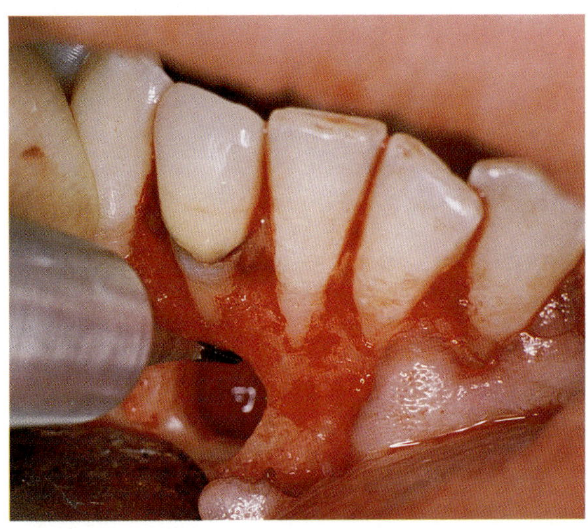

- Beveled, monoplane resection:
  - 45-degree angle
  - encompasses apical third
  - unobstructed visualization

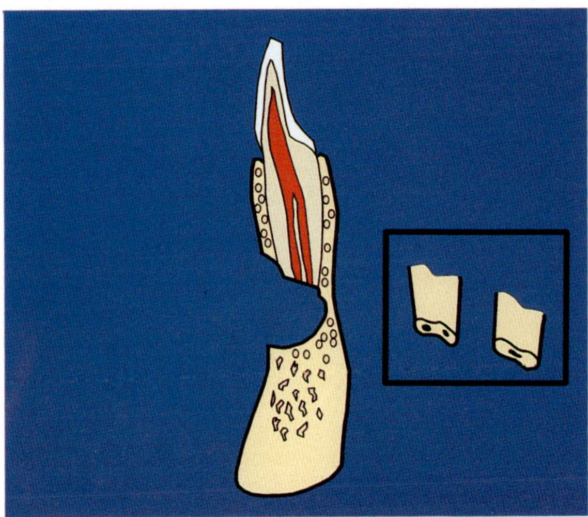

- Resected root of mandibular incisor.

Apical Preparation

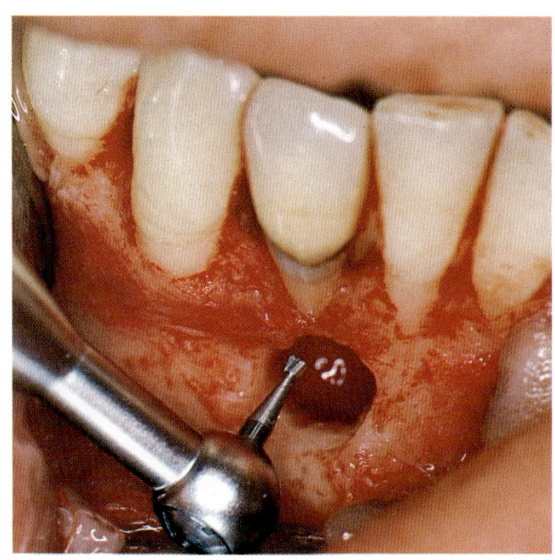

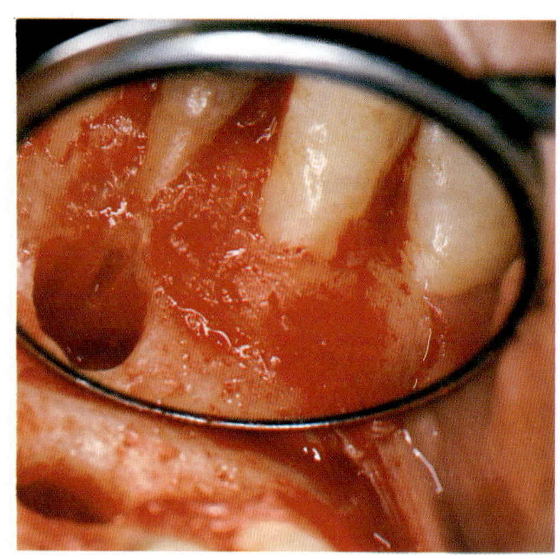

- Class I:
  - one-canal system
- Undercut slot:
  - two-canal system

Apical Isolation

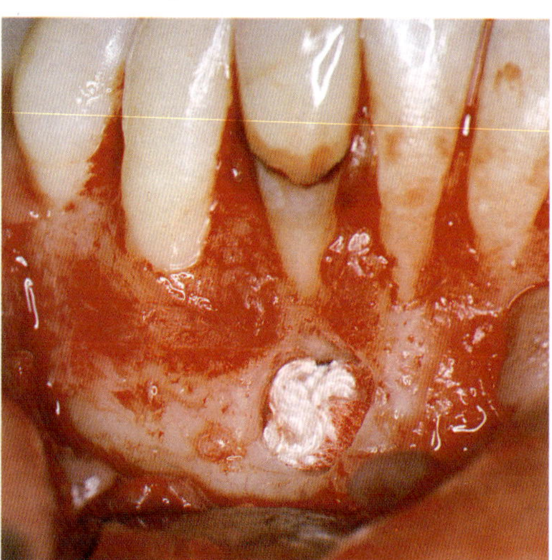

- Control hemorrhage with:
  - *Nu Gauze*
  - bone wax
  - *Gelfoam*
  - *Surgicel*
- Dry apical preparation with modified paper points.

Retrograde Obturation

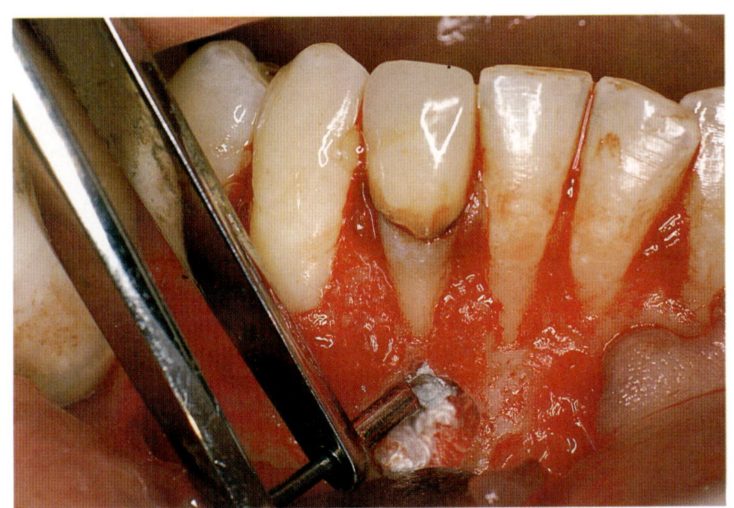

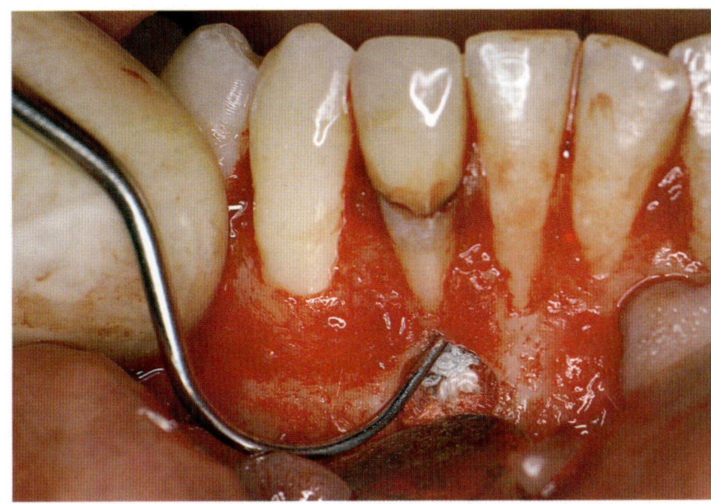

- Choose material:
  - amalgam
  - *IRM* (Intermediate Restorative Material)
- Use minicarrier.
- Use modified condenser.

Radiographic Confirmation

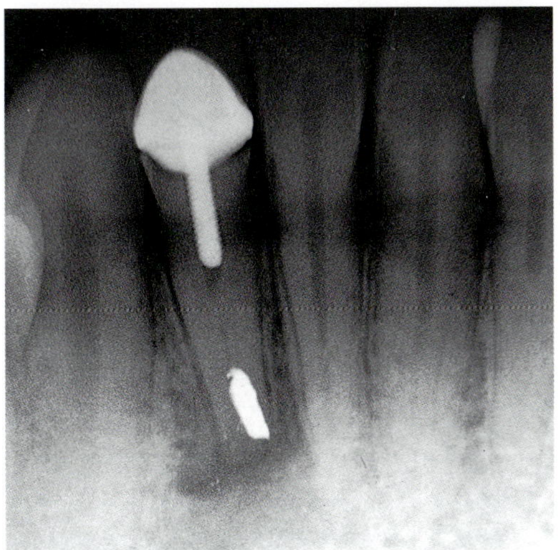

- Take radiograph before closure.
- Inspect for:
  - complete resection
  - retrograde filling alignment
  - retrograde filling debris
- Remove hemorrhage control packing before final closure.

Final Closure

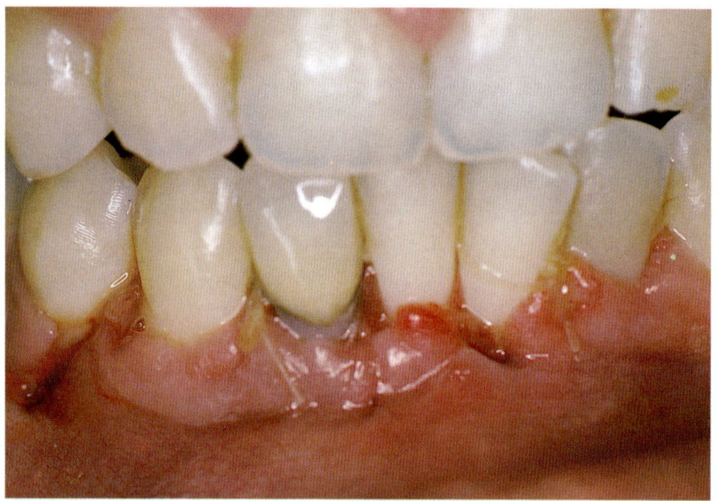

- Use single suspensory suture around involved tooth.
- Use interrupted sutures interproximally and along vertical incision, as needed.

Surgical Followup

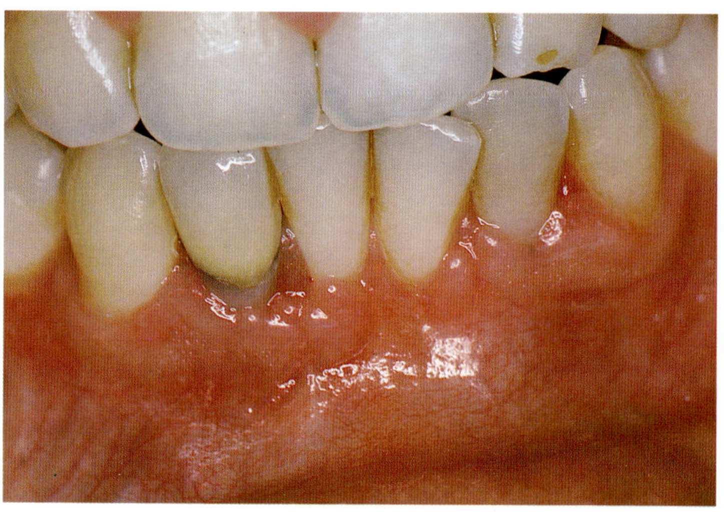

- Monitor patient for:
  - tissue readaptation
  - healing
  - oral hygiene

10 Mandibular Molar Surgery

Some of the contended contraindications for mandibular molar surgery are: thick cortical bone, the presence of the mandibular canal and mental foramen, buttressed bone, and the external oblique ridge. For the most part, these are easily dealt with using the newer technology that is presently available. Some of the newer advances include: high-torque surgical handpieces for bone removal and root resection; fiberoptics for enhanced illumination of the surgical field; and optical magnification for increased clinical visualization. Visualization of the shape, size, and morphology of the mandibular roots plays an important role in the planning of any surgical procedure. The probability of anomalies and variations is always present.

The pyramidal projection of buccal bone and the thickness of the external oblique ridge as it progresses distally are frequently good indicators of the degree of surgical difficulty. The clinician must be aware of this when considering molar surgery on the distal root of the mandibular first molar as well as the roots of the second mandibular molar. Anatomic variation will at times limit access to some mandibular molars.

In most instances, the mandibular neurovascular bundle is inferior and lingual to the mesial root of the mandibular first molar. It progresses buccally and superiorly as it travels distally. The buccal lingual position of the neurovascular bundle relative to the roots of the mandibular molar roots is of great importance. A technique to demonstrate this relationship is based on the vertical angulation of the radiograph:

1. An initial parallel radiograph is taken.
2. The patient's head and film position remain constant.
3. A second film is directed upward at an angle of (−)25 degrees.
4. A comparison of both radiographs is made.
5. If the mandibular canal is buccal to the molar roots, it will appear to move upward.
6. Conversely, if the mandibular canal is on the lingual aspect of the roots, it will appear to move downward.

A panoramic radiograph is an excellent adjunct for an overall view of both the mandibular canal and the mental foramen and their relationship to the root apices. The panoramic radiograph also affords the practitioner the opportunity to observe large lesions in their entirety and compare the contralateral side for similar pathologies.

Whenever surgery is considered in the mandibular posterior region, the position of the mental foramen must be identified. Generally, the position of the mental foramen ranges in location from apically between the first and second premolars to directly below the apex of the second premolar. Radiographic confirmation of the mental foramen can be determined on panoramic radiographs.

The likelihood of paresthesias, although minimal, is possible when endodontic surgery is performed on mandibular teeth. Both the mental foramen and the mandibular neurovascular bundle can be involved. Patients are always informed of this possibility before surgery. If a paresthesia occurs, it is generally of short duration and resolves uneventfully.

A thorough understanding of the soft tissue and muscle attachments in the mandibular posterior region is essential for developing the basic principles of flap design. Improved access to the cortical bone in the area of the surgical site depends on our knowledge of soft tissue limitations, bony anatomy, and muscle attachments in both the premolar and molar areas. They have a direct bearing on the design of the flap, tissue replacement, suturing, and healing.

Surgical technique notes

Flap design

The mucoperiosteal triangular flap with a distal relaxing incision is used most often.

Incision

The mental foramen sets the parameters for the anterior extent of the vertical incision, which is placed either at the mesial-buccal line angle of the first premolar or at the distal-buccal line angle of the canine. The vertical incision should be directed straight downward and not angled. This is to avoid the prominent eminence of the canine. Inclusion of the papilla in the flap again depends on the position of the mental foramen and muscle attachments. A relaxing incision, usually made at the distal aspect of the second molar, facilitates reflection and avoids tissue tears and forced extension of the flap.

Flap reflection

As previously described, the no. 4 Molt curet with its broad, sharp, convex surface is ideal for initial reflection; in contrast, the no. 9 periosteal elevator with its pointed end, when used interproximally, tends to crush the fragile interseptal bone. Use undermining elevation, starting at the midpoint of the vertical incision and directing the reflection distally and superiorly until the distal relaxing incision is reached. Buttressed bone with its irregular contours presents some difficulty when reflecting the flap. If the flap is not supported with a quartered 2 × 2 gauze as the reflection progresses distally, an inadequate reflection, leaving periosteum behind, may occur. There is also an increased possibility of slipping and perforating the flap. Failure to make a complete and clean reflection of the periosteum will result in postoperative bleeding, swelling, pain, and delayed healing.

Flap retraction

As the flap is retracted, take care in the region of the premolars. Occasionally the neurovascular bundle of the mental foramen may be visualized. When this occurs, place the retractor above the bundle and perpendicular to bone; this prevents damage to the neurovascular bundle and at the same time facilitates flap retraction.

Cortical bone removal

Pathologic fenestrations of the cortical bone overlying mandibular molars is not common. *Never begin cortical bone removal where you think the apex is.* Use the rule of thirds and any root contour present to direct your initial bone removal. Start in the mid-third of the root area and progress apically. First remove cortical bone over the root, then use the root as a guide until the apical area is defined. The mid-third of the root is visualized along with the apex in an ovoid-type preparation, giving the required visibility. Remove pathologic tissue and submit it for biopsy.

Root resection

Never resect a root that is not defined with an apex that cannot be seen. Adequate access to the root is essential. Lingual plate perforation can be avoided when the root is visualized and the root defined. Make sure the resection is not horizontal but is angled for visualization, apical preparation, and placement of the retrograde materials. Using a fissure bur in a surgical handpiece, make a continuous, clean, and sharp cut. The root can be prepared with either a slot or a Class I preparation to receive the retrograde filling material of choice.

Apical preparation

Although the mesial root is broad in its buccal-lingual dimension, difficulty can be encountered if the angulation of the resection is too flat. A beveled, broad cut surface presents with excellent visibility and reveals canals and/or an isthmus. Use a microhandpiece to prepare a Class I or a slot preparation to receive the retrograde material. If a slot is used, place the fissure bur flat on the root's beveled surface. Then prepare the slot as the bur is withdrawn buccally; this will prevent perforation of the lingual surface of the root and the lingual cortical plate.

Retrograde obturation

Place the hemorrhage-control packing in the prepared surgical site. This packing also acts as a physical barrier for retrograde filling debris. Place the retrograde obturation material of choice and remove excess debris with copious irrigation and suction. Remove the packing and take a confirmation radiograph before final closure.

Final closure

Place a single suspensory suture around the surgically involved tooth. Use interrupted sutures interproximally and along the vertical incisions, as needed.

Followup

The patient is seen 3 to 5 days after surgery to monitor soft tissue healing, evaluate for any paresthesia, and remove sutures (if not absorbable).

Mandibular Molar Surgery

Posterior Mandible

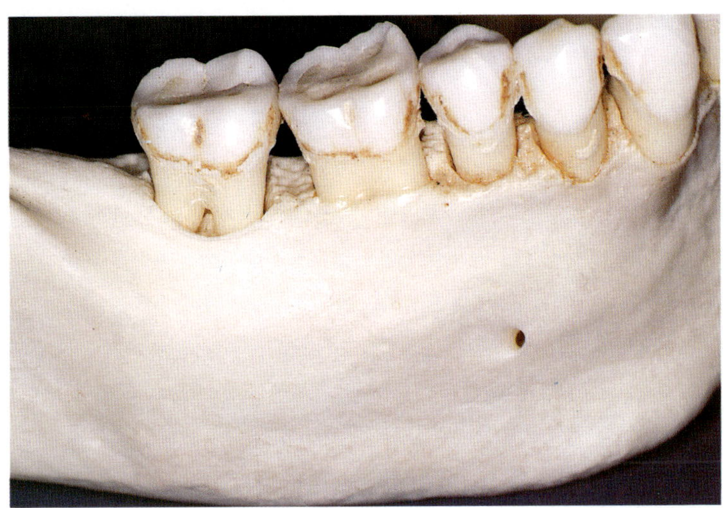

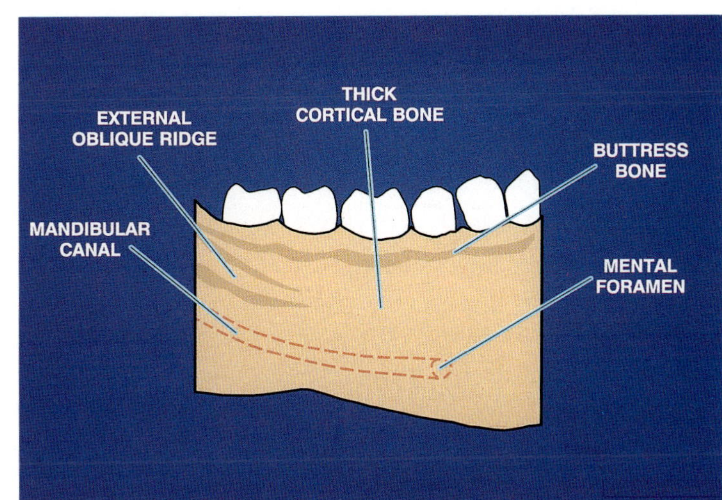

- Thick cortical bone.
- Mandibular canal.
- Mental foramen.
- Buttress bone.
- External oblique ridge.

Root Anatomy

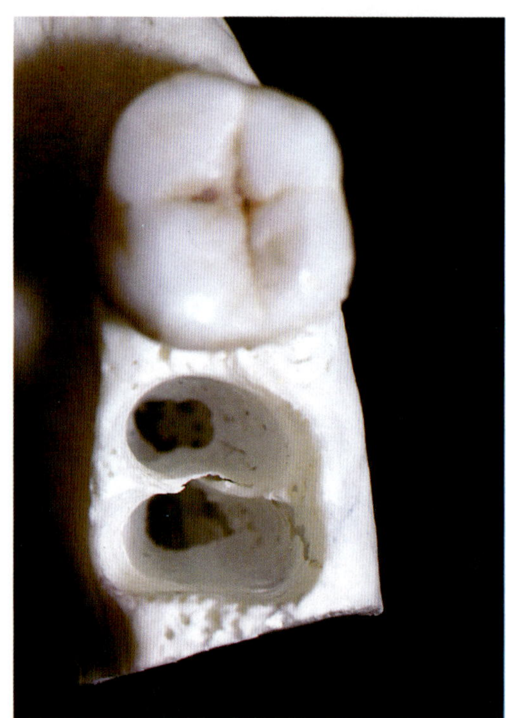

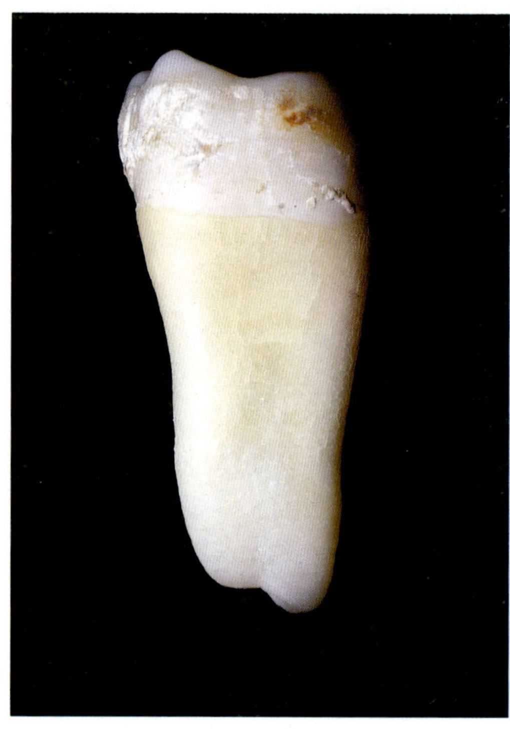

Mesial Root:

- Broad buccal-lingual dimension.
- Oval, kidney shaped, figure-eight.
- Vertical to distal angulation.
- Root length determined radiographically.
- Buccal and lingual canals may vary in length.

Distal Root:

- Oval, conical cross section.
- Distal angulation.
- Thicker cortical bone.
- Root length determined radiographically.
- May have two canals.

Pyramidal Projection

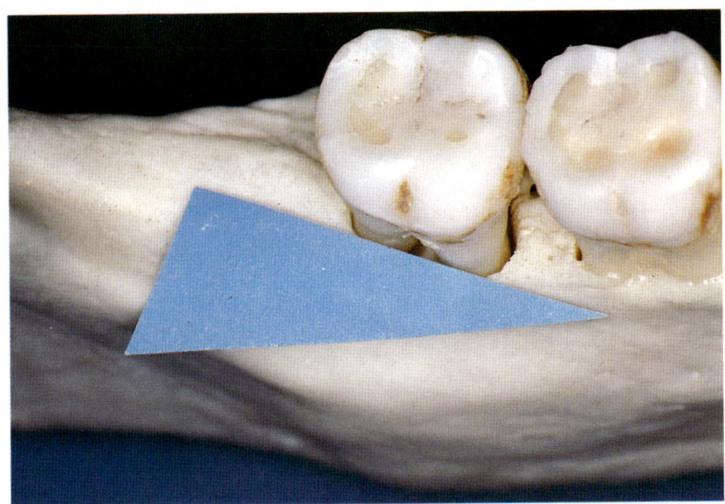

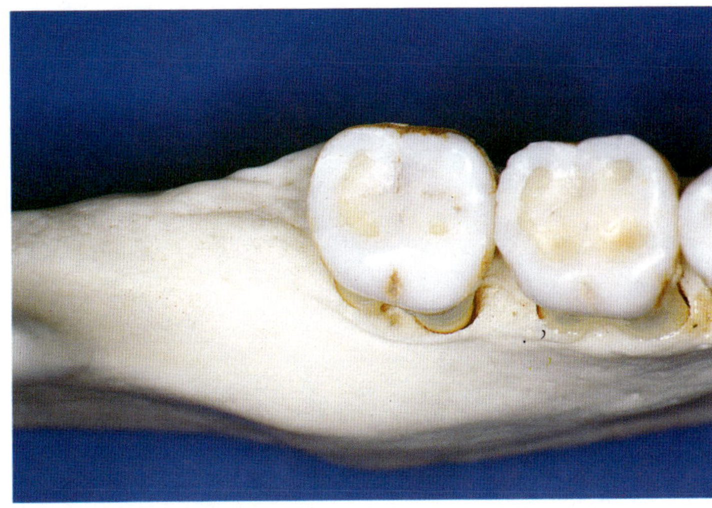

- Thickness of buccal cortical bone increases posteriorly.

Mandibular Canal

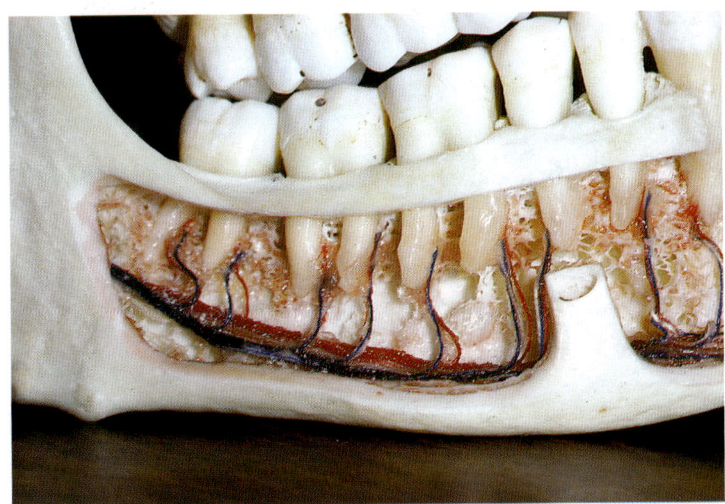

- Proximity to root apices.
- Position of mental foramen.

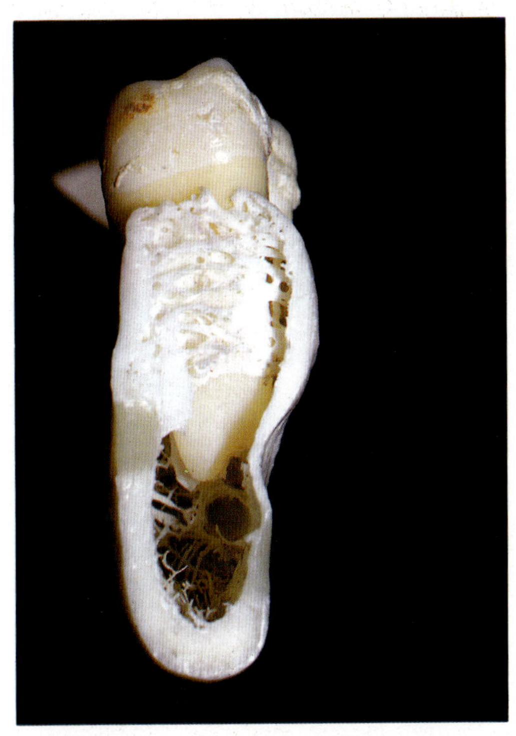

- Lingual and inferior position of the mandibular canal in relation to the first molar.

Mandibular Vestibule (Narrow) (N)

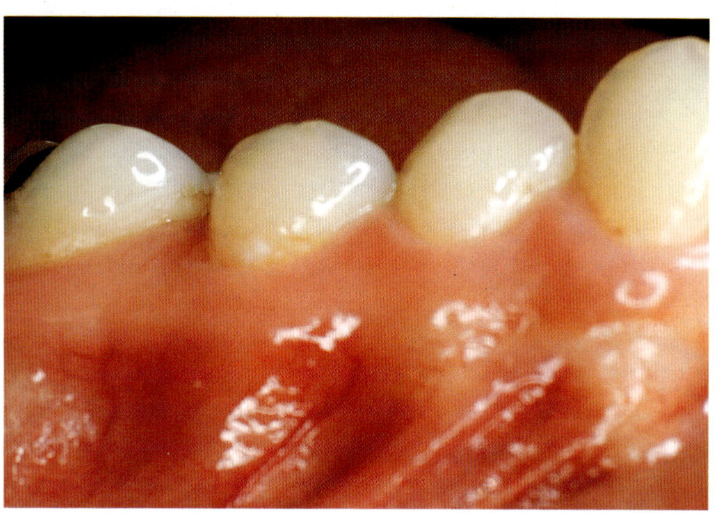

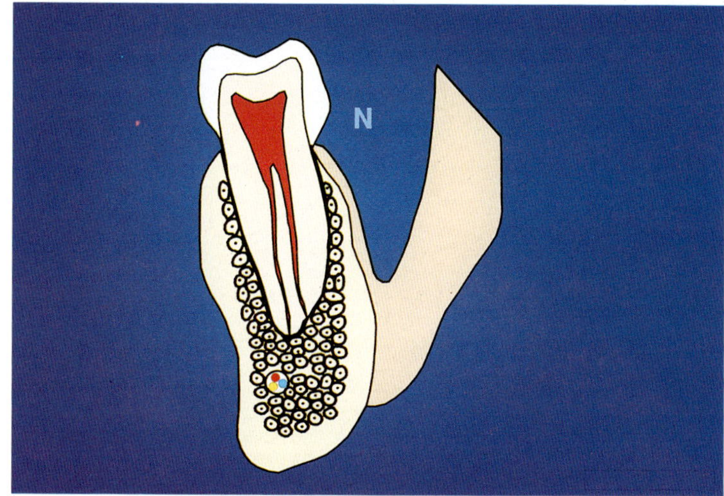

- Greater surgical access.
- Diminished amounts of buccal bone.
- Conducive to healing because of low muscle attachments and adequate attached gingiva.

Mandibular Vestibule (Shallow) (S)

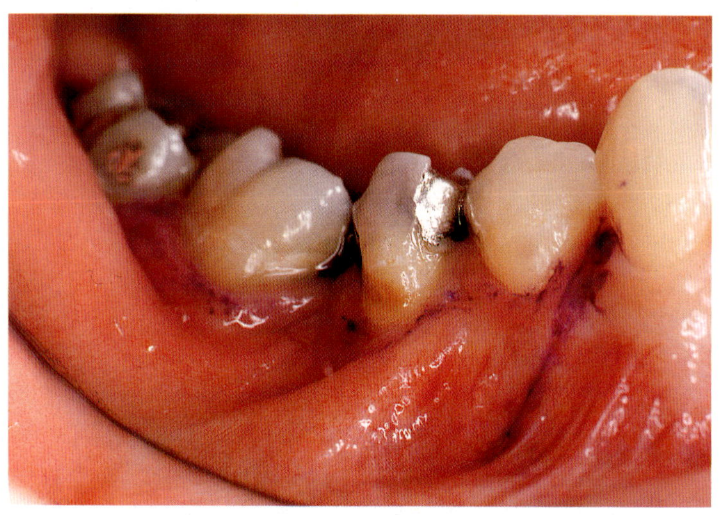

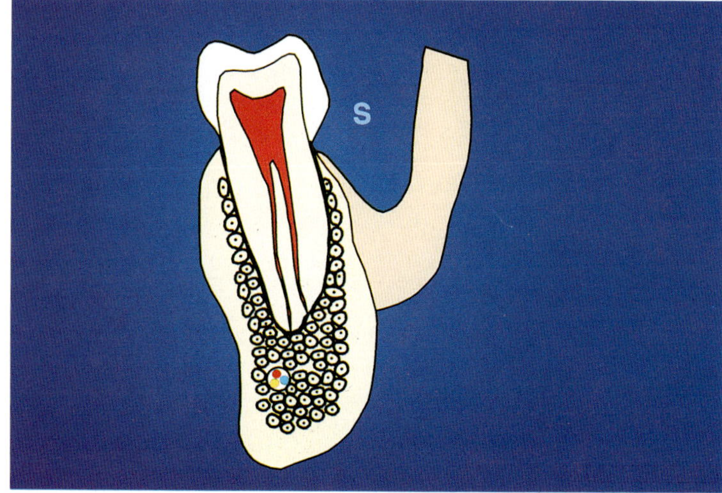

- Limited surgical access.
- Accompanied by thicker cortical bone.
- Decreased healing potential because of high muscle attachments and minimal attached gingiva.

Mesial Root Mandibular First Molar (Apical Surgery)

Soft Tissue Anatomy

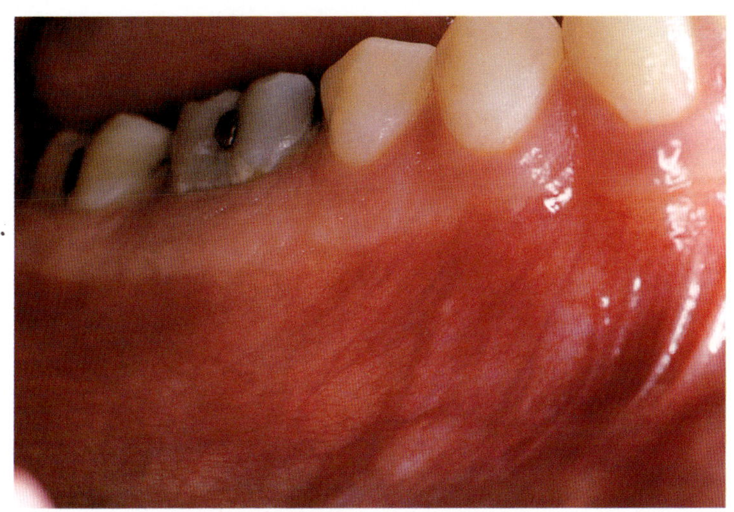

- Narrow vestibule.
- Low muscle attachments.
- Adequate width of attached gingiva.

Diagnostic Radiographs

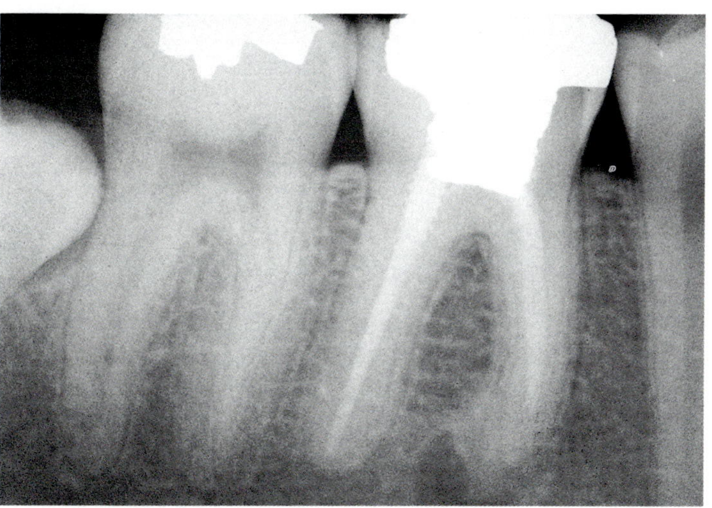

- Straight-on and parallel views show:
  - — length and shape of roots
  - — inclination of roots
- Mesial shift detects:
  - — unfilled canals
  - — root anomalies
- Panoramic view shows:
  - — relative position of mandibular canal and mental foramen

Mucoperiosteal Flap (Triangular)

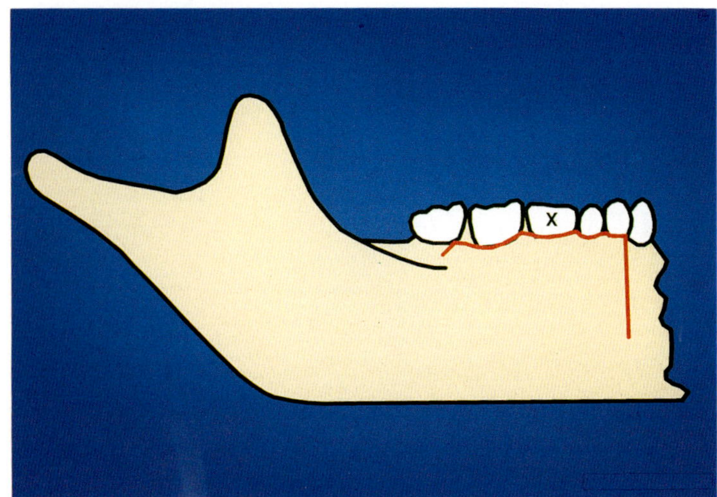

- Horizontal incision:
  —distal relaxing incision
- Vertical incision.

Surgical Geography

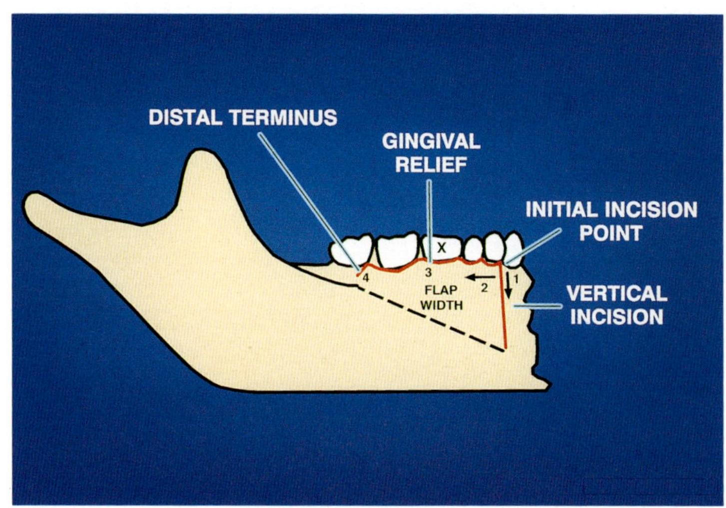

- Initial incision point.
- Vertical incision.
- Gingival relief.
- Distal terminus.

Mental Foramen — Position Sets the Parameter for the Vertical Incision*

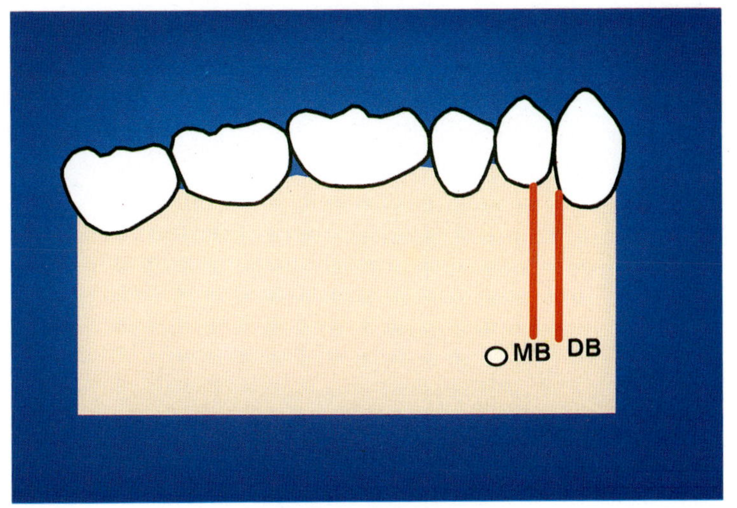

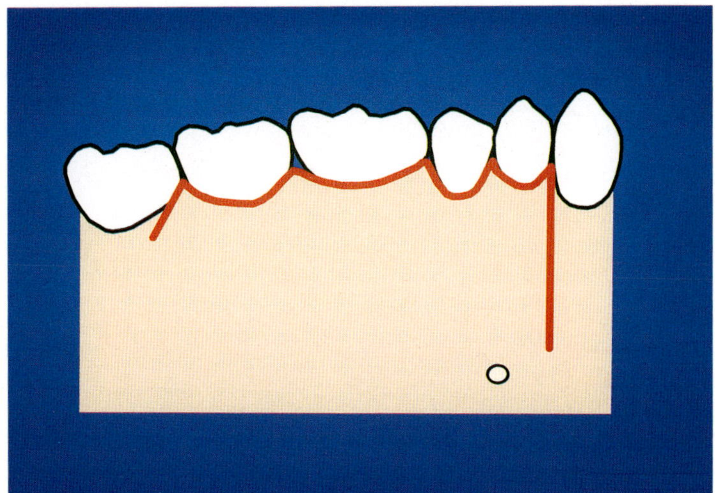

- **MB,** mesial buccal.
- **DB,** distal buccal.

Location	*Mastuda (329 mandibles)* Left %	*Mastuda (329 mandibles)* Right %	*Tebo and Telford (100 mandibles)* Left %	*Tebo and Telford (100 mandibles)* Right %	*Sweet (585 patients)* %	*Present study (1,000 patients)* Left %	*Present study (1,000 patients)* Right %
Mesial to the first premolar	–	–	–	–	2.5	2.1	0.9
Apical area of first premolar	0.9	5.5	1.2	2.3	7.9	2.9	3.5
Between the two premolars	11.3	20.7	20.4	25.3	63.3	72.6	68.1
Apical area of second premolar	69.9	67.2	52.8	46.0	22.9	17.2	20.7
Distal to the second premolar	17.9	6.6	25.6	26.4	3.4	5.2	6.8

*Fishel D, Buchner A, Hershkowith A, Kaffe I. Roentgenologic study of the mental foramen. *Oral Surg* 1976; 41: 682-686.

Determining Position for Vertical Incision

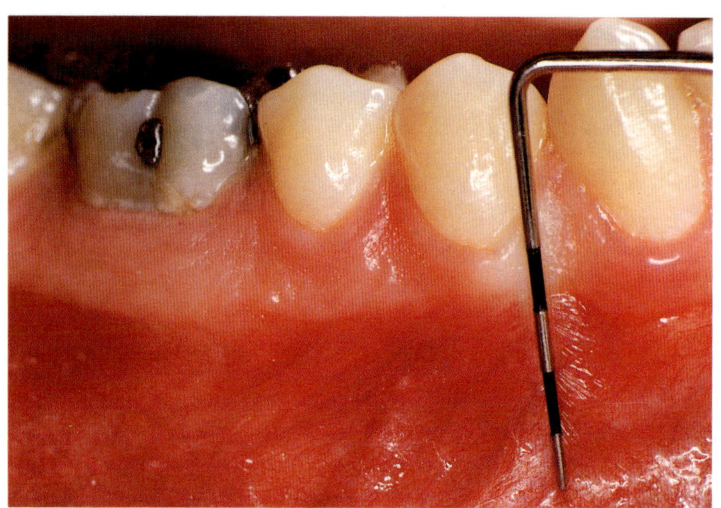

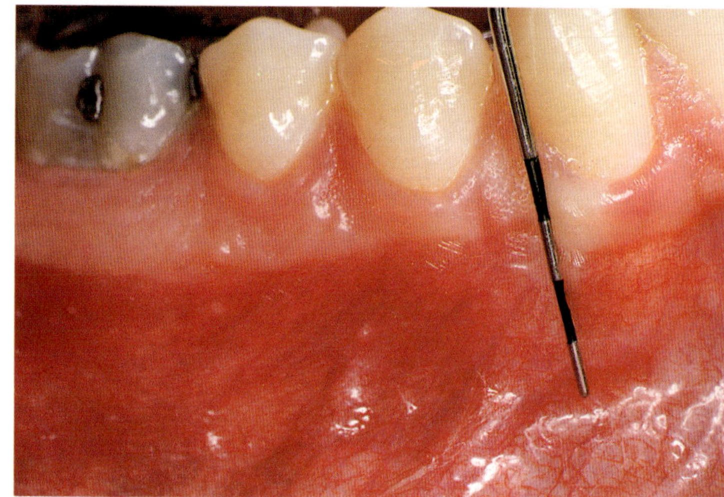

- Mesial buccal line angle of the first premolar.
- Distal buccal line angle of the canine.

Vertical Incision

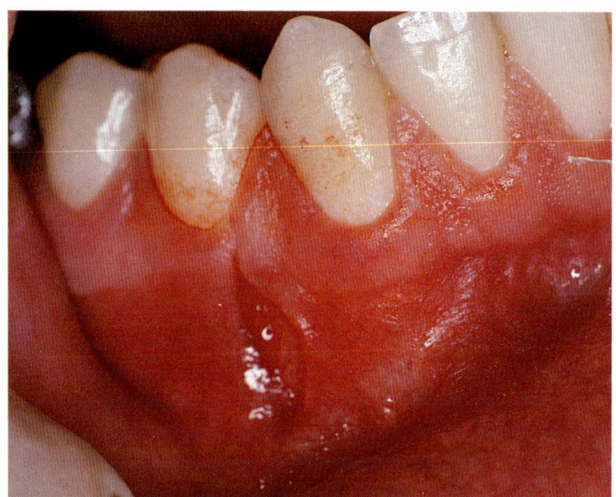

- Extends into vestibular mucosa.
- Full extent depends on:
  - depth of vestibule
  - position of mental foramen
  - access required

Horizontal Incision

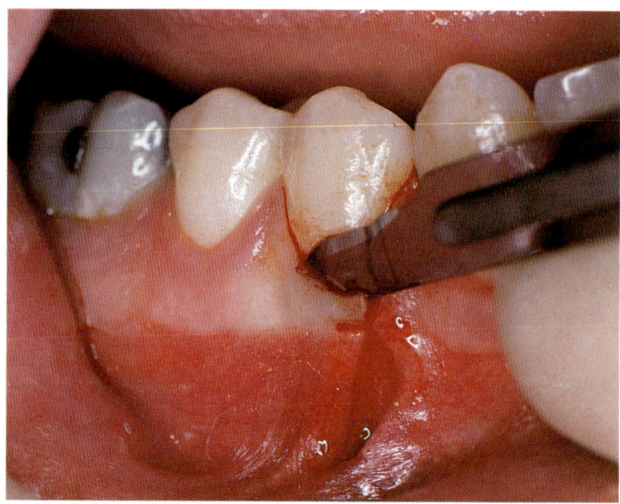

- Intrasulcular.
- Separates periodontal attachment from the teeth at the level of crestal bone.
- Use interproximal tooth surface as guide for the blade.
- Separation of papillary region in the col (mid-papilla) allows buccal papilla to be reflected with the flap.

Flap Design Completed

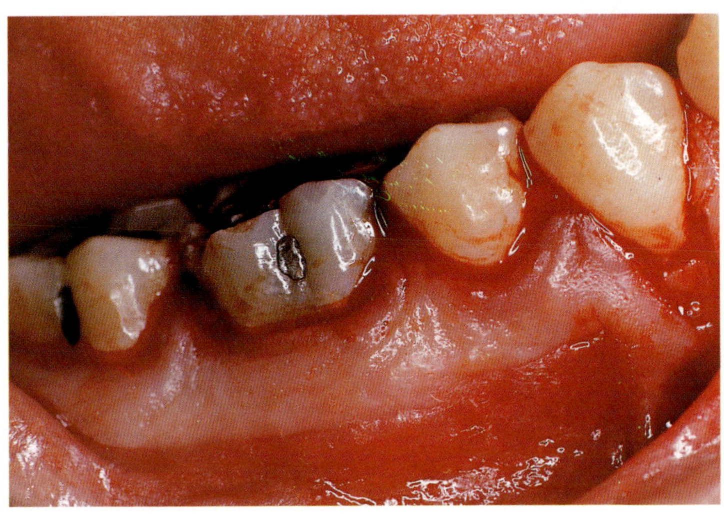

- Incision through periosteum to bone.
- Intrasulcular tissue is loose and freely moveable.

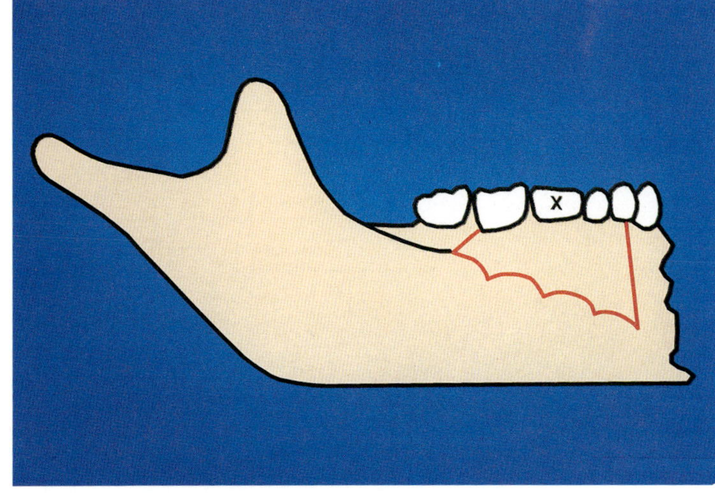

- Horizontal and vertical incisions completed.

Flap Reflection

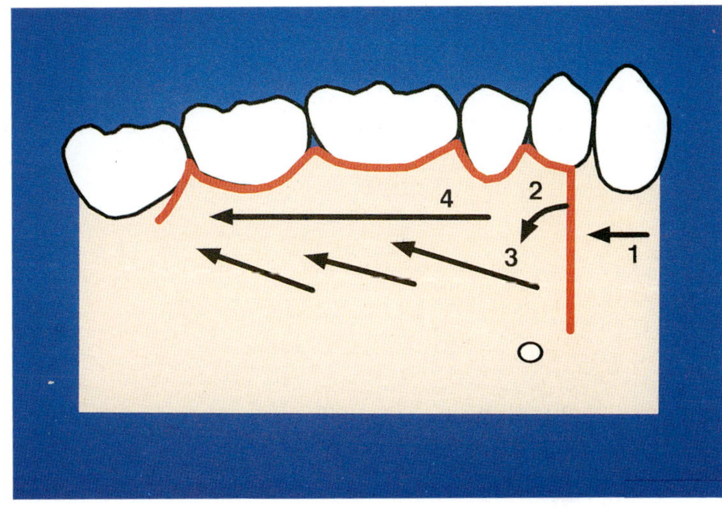

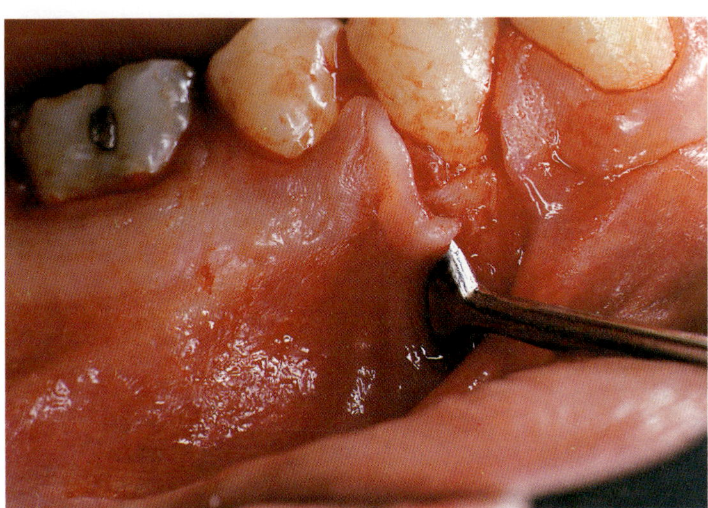

- Begin at mid-vertical incision, apply pressure superiorly.
- Free papilla.
- Complete release of vertical incision.
- Complete posterior extent of flap by applying pressure posteriorly and superiorly.

Reflection and Flap Support

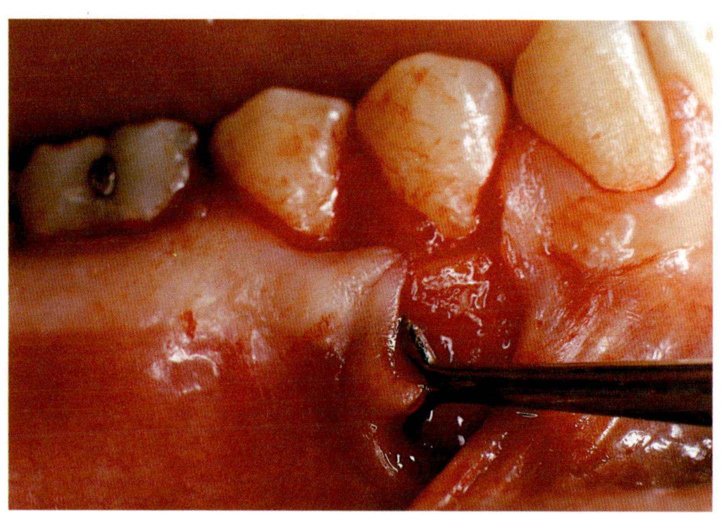

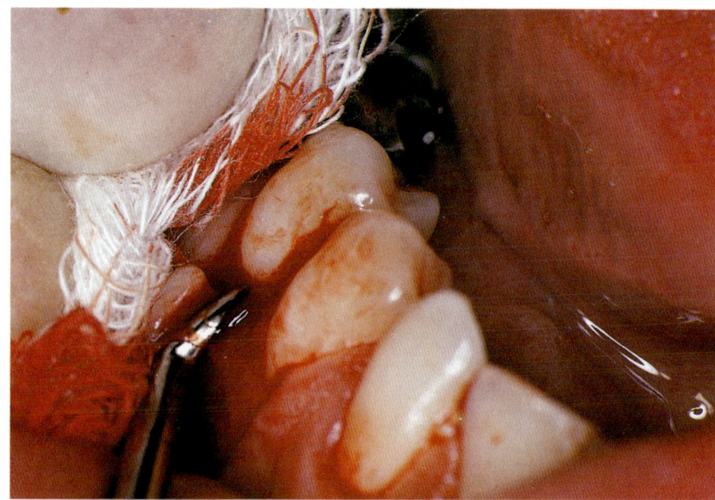

- Buttress bone reflection:
  — compression support with gauze
  — prevents flap perforation due to irregular bony architecture
  — atraumatic reflection of periosteum and superficial tissue

Rule of Thirds (Visualize Surgical Geography)

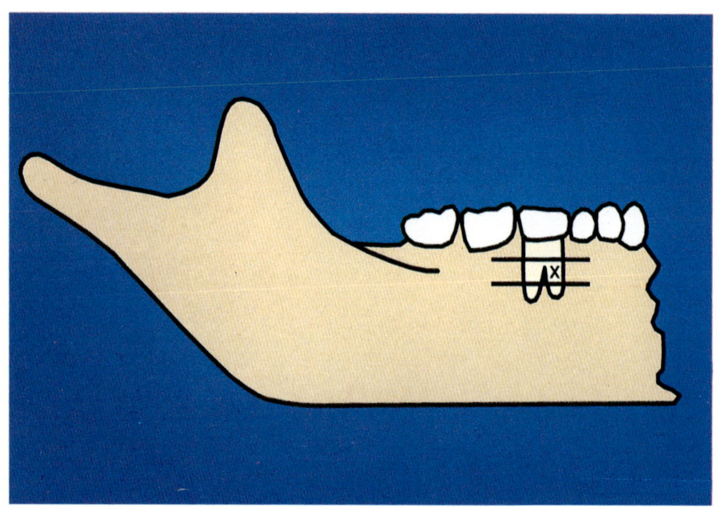

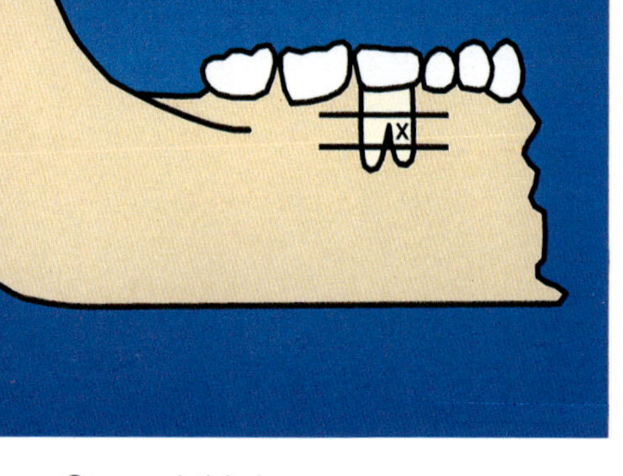

- Coronal third.
- Middle third.
- Apical third.

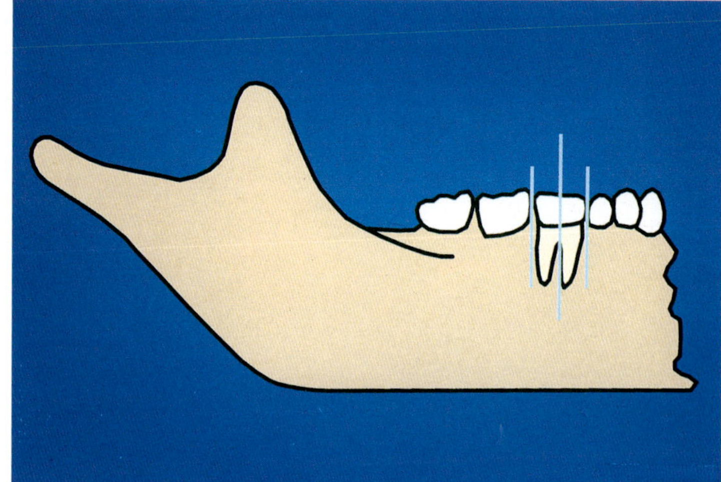

- Mesial third.
- Furcal third.
- Distal third.

Placement for Initial Cortical Bone Removal

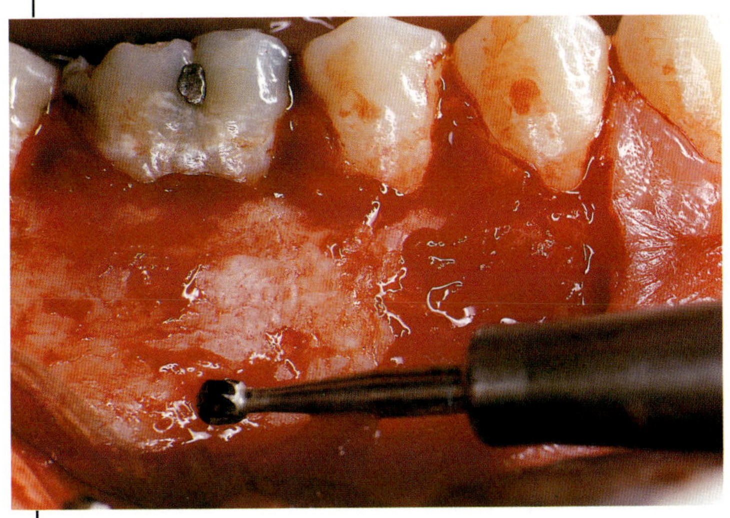

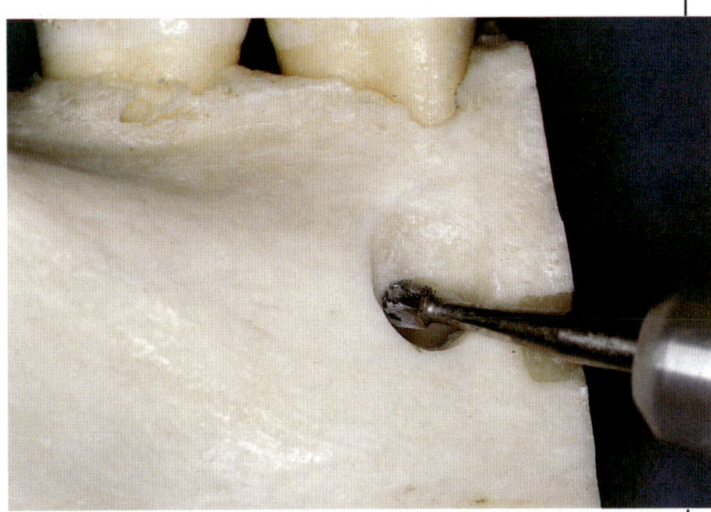

- Avoid an apical start:
  - use root eminence when present
  - for the mesial root, begin in the middle and mesial third
  - remove bone until root is exposed
  - use root as a guide to the apex

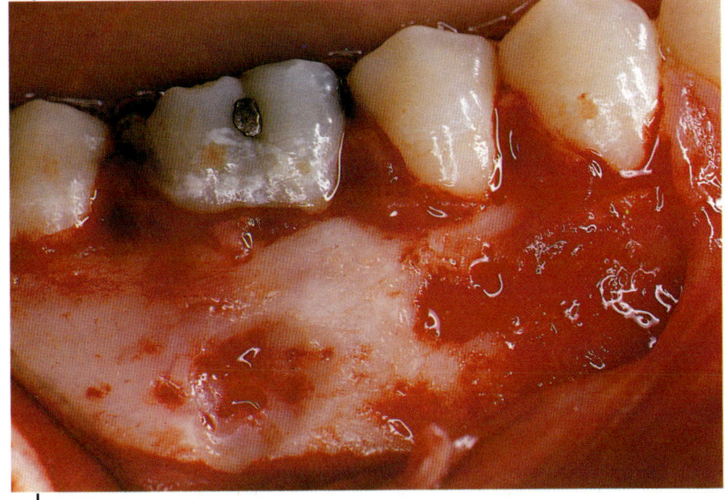

- Initial bone removal.

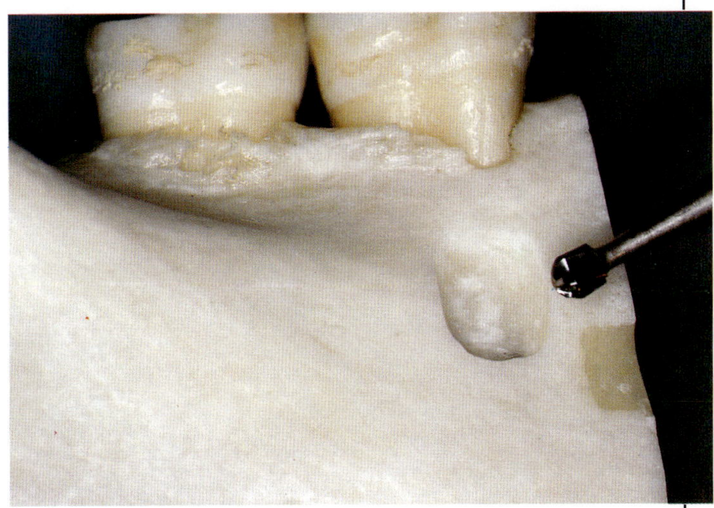

- Cortical/medullary bone penetration.

Bone Removal — Root Access

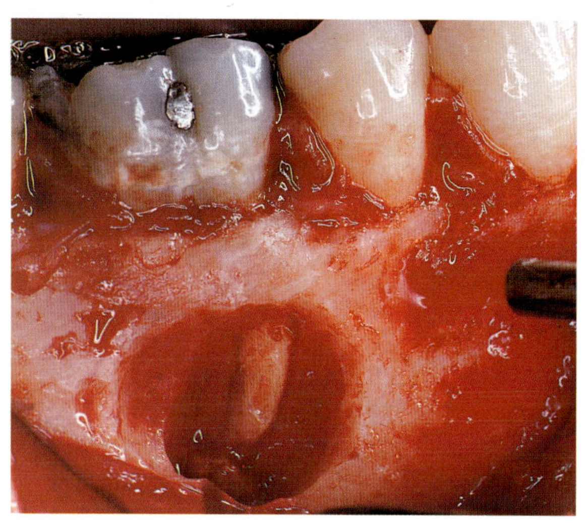

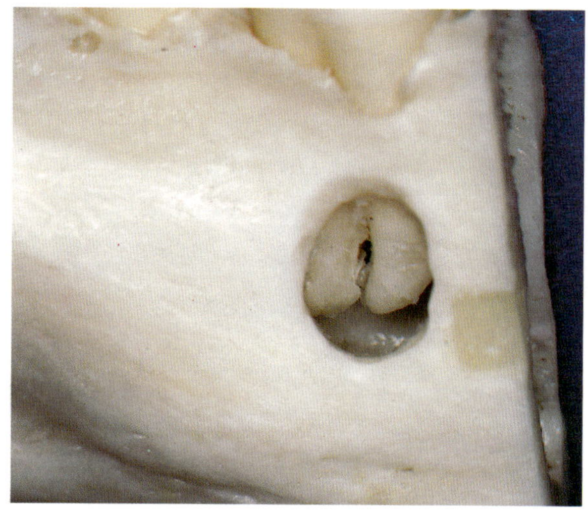

- Apical localization.
- Define mesial-distal and buccal-lingual boundaries.

Root Resection

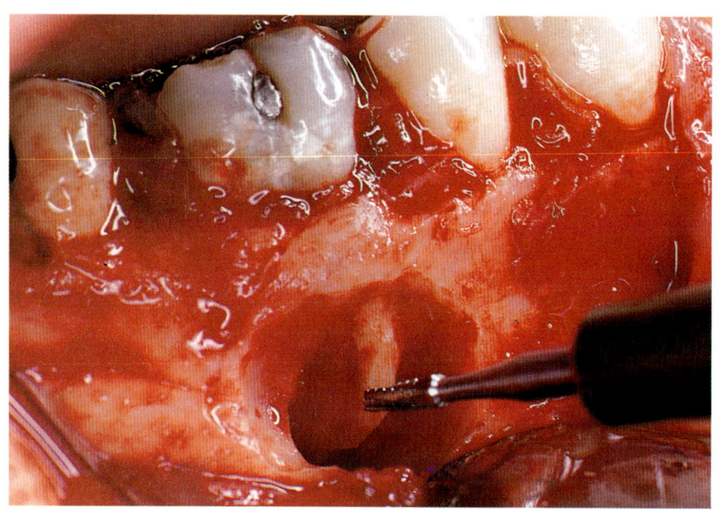

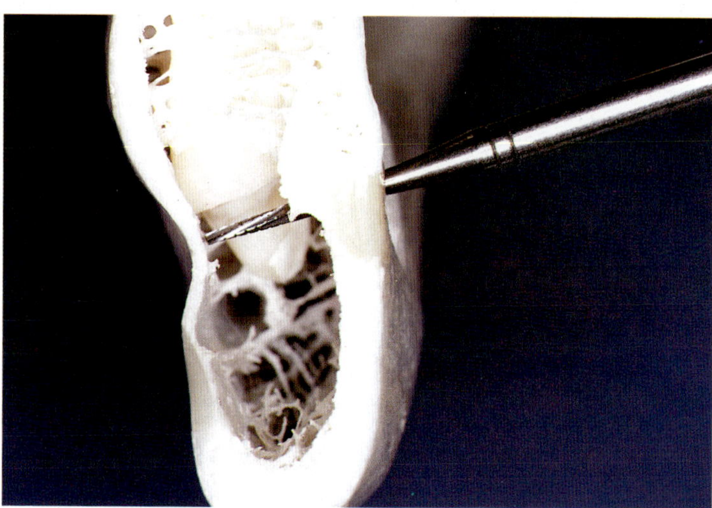

- Begin at junction of middle and apical third.
- 45-degree angle.
- Resect definitely and completely.

Resected Root

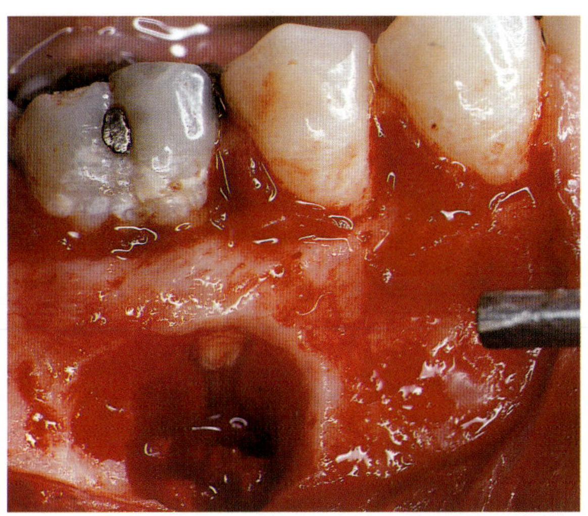

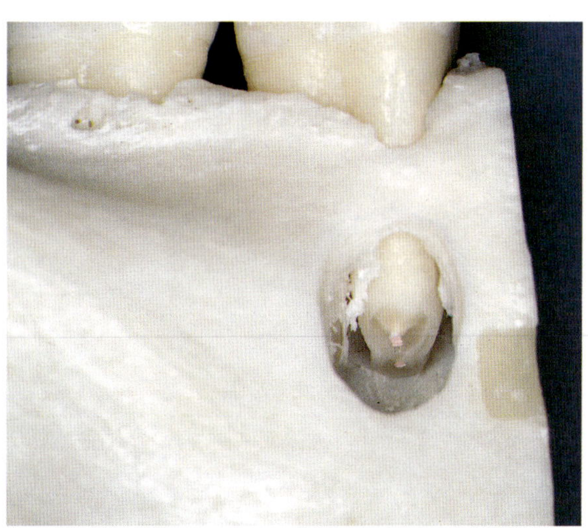

- Complete resection.
- Angle allows visualization of canals and isthmus.
- Visualization of periodontal ligament and root contour.

Adequate Surgical Access and Complete Resection

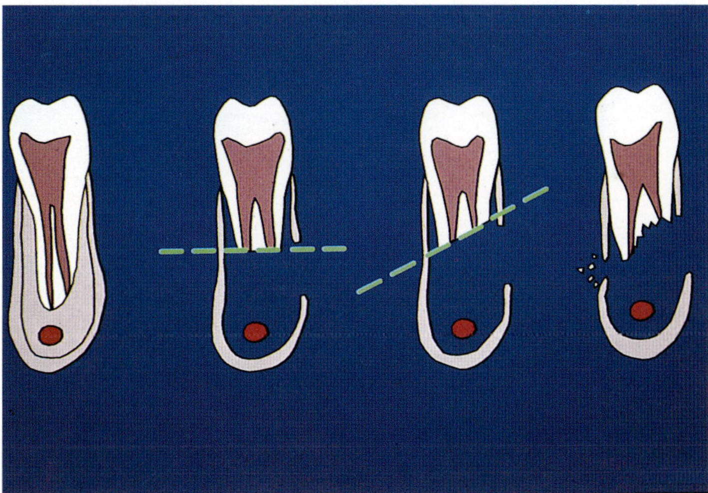

- Avoids irregular apical cuts.
- Avoids lingual plate perforation.
- Avoids horizontal cuts, which limit apical visualization.

Apical Preparation — Class I

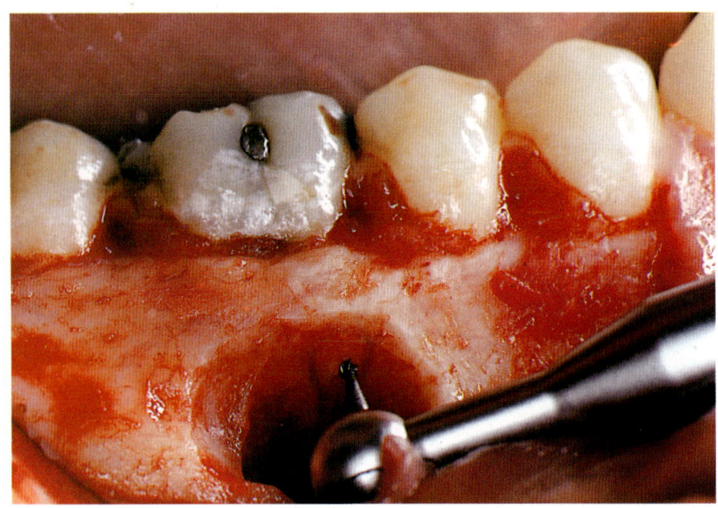

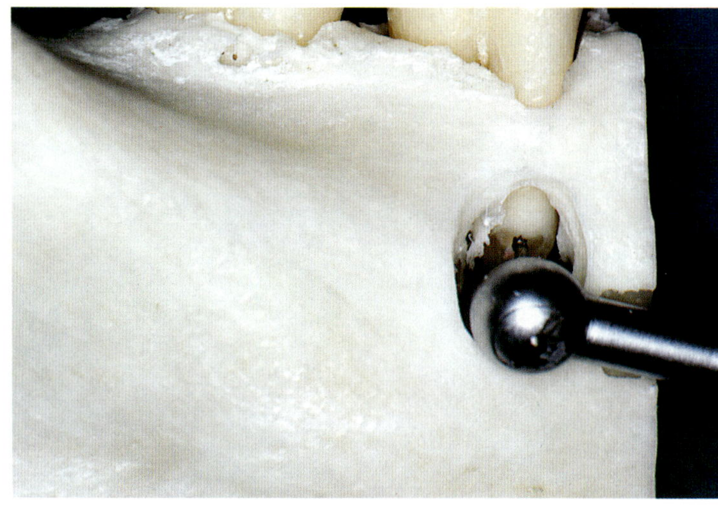

- Use microhandpiece.
- Class I preparation vertically within the canal space.

Apical Preparation — Slot

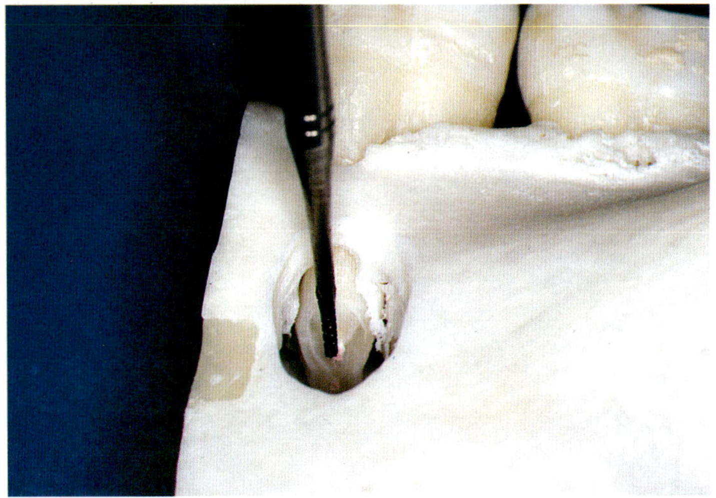

- Inspect furcal concavity before preparation.
- Use straight handpiece and fissure bur.
- Use when isthmus is patent.
- Position bur in line with orifices and at angle of root resection.

Slot Preparation with *IRM*

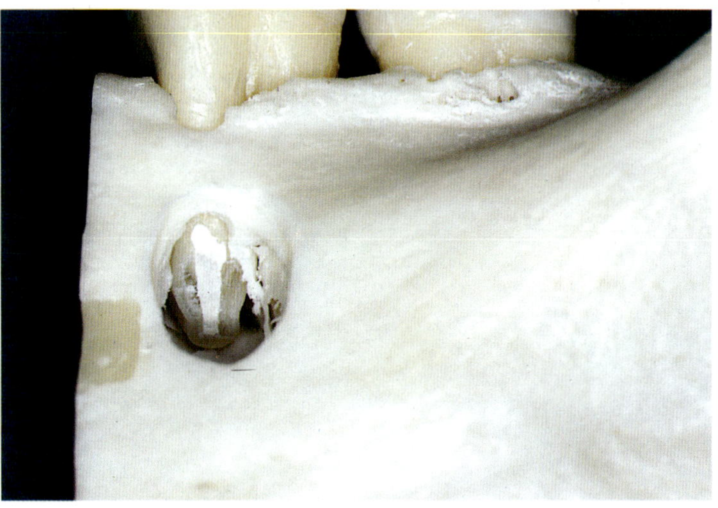

- Easy to handle and place
- Sealing ability is within accepted standards.
- Biologic compatibility is within accepted standards.
- Can be used when metal posts are present in the canal.

Retrograde Obturation

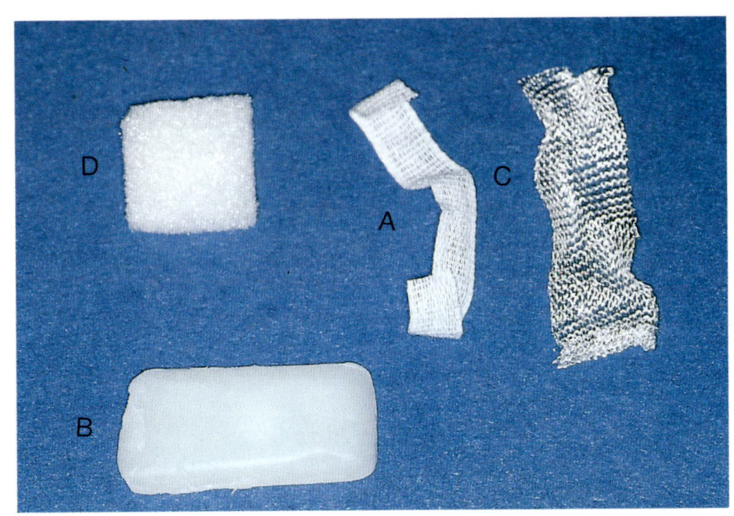

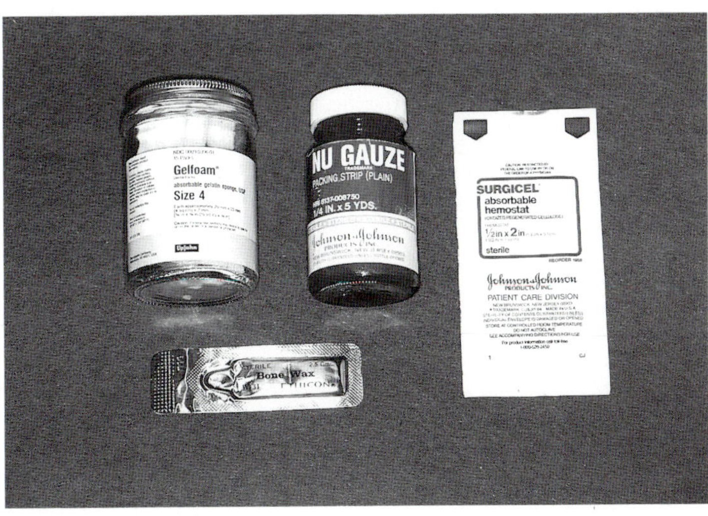

- Isolate for hemorrhage control and apical splatter with:
  - A, *Nu Gauze*
  - B, bone wax
  - C, *Surgicel*
  - D, *Gelfoam*

Drying Retrograde Preparation

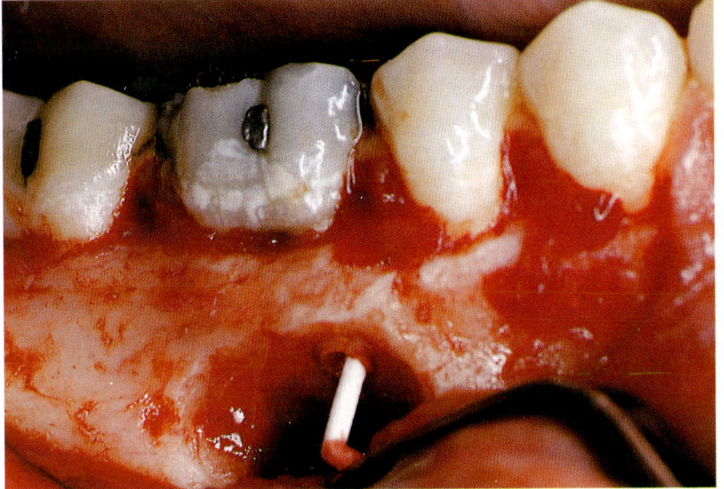

- Use cut end of paper points held with cotton pliers.
- Dried preparation is then ready for retrofilling.

Placement of Retrofilling

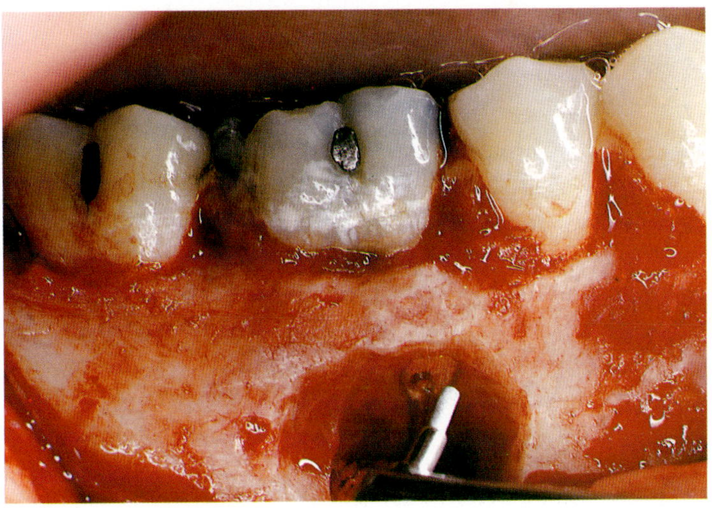

- Use miniamalgam carrier; it allows for placement in confined areas.

Clinical View of Class I Retrofill

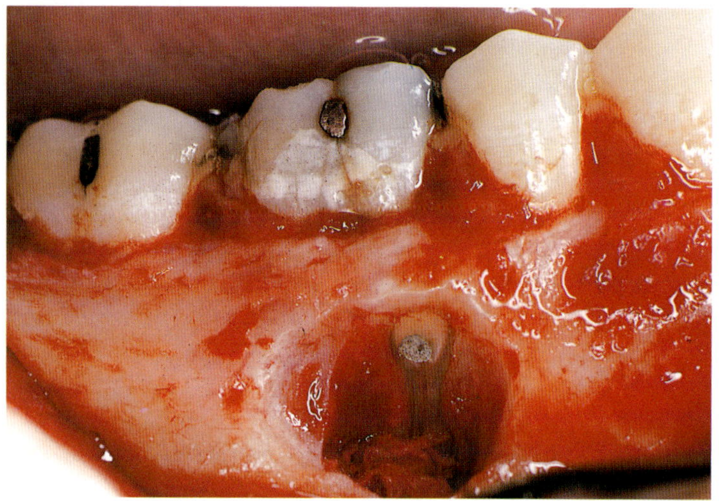

- Extremely narrow and sclerosed isthmus precludes slot preparation.

Slot Preparation with Amalgam

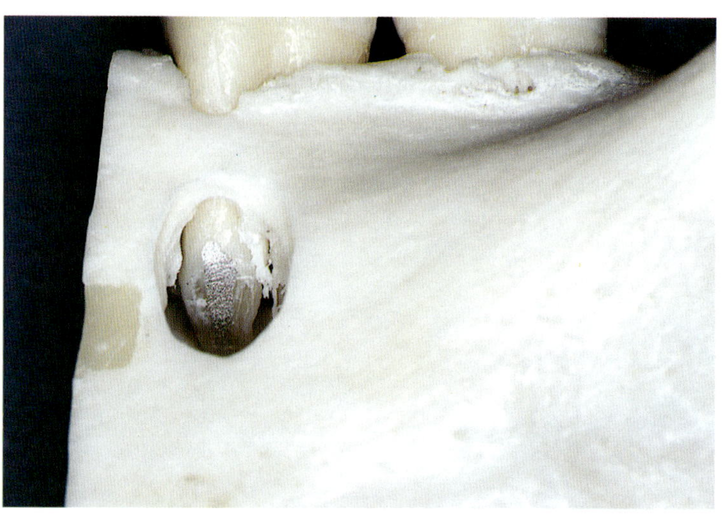

- Amalgam is used by most clinicians because:
  - it is time proven
  - its sealing ability is within accepted standards

Radiographic View of Retrofill

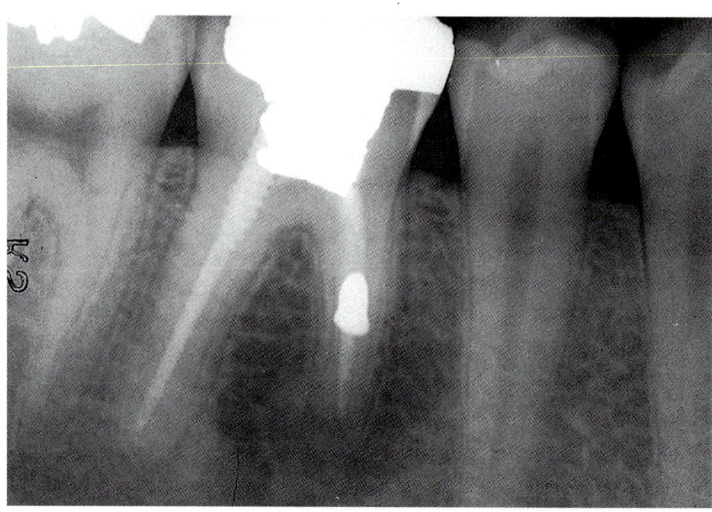

- Obtain radiograph before wound closure to verify complete root resection and retrofilling placement.
- Check for apical debris.

Wound Closure

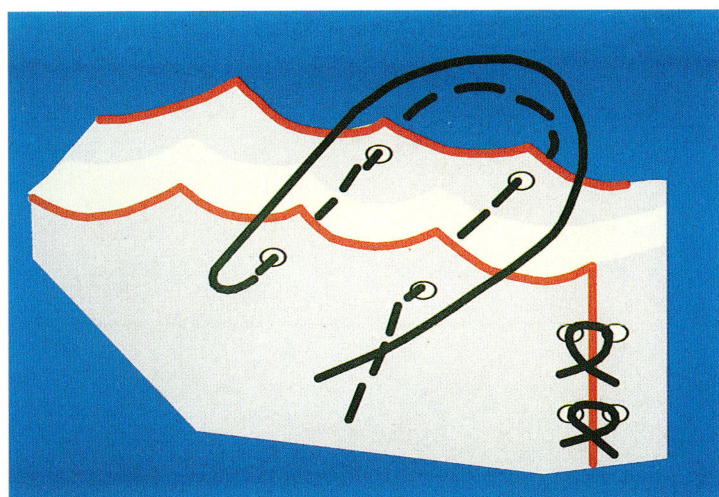

- Remove hemorrhage-control packing before closure.
- Irrigate copiously before closure.
- Reposition flap — 5-minutes' pressure with gauze.
- Have assistant apply gauze pressure during suturing.
- Apply pressure for 5 minutes after suturing.

Immediate Postsurgical Appearance

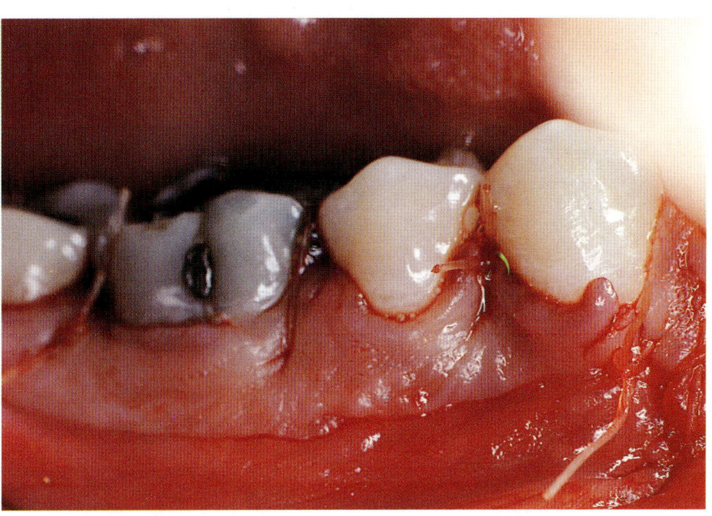

- Use single suspensory suture on surgically involved tooth.
- Use interrupted sutures interproximally and on vertical incision, as needed.

Postsurgical Followup

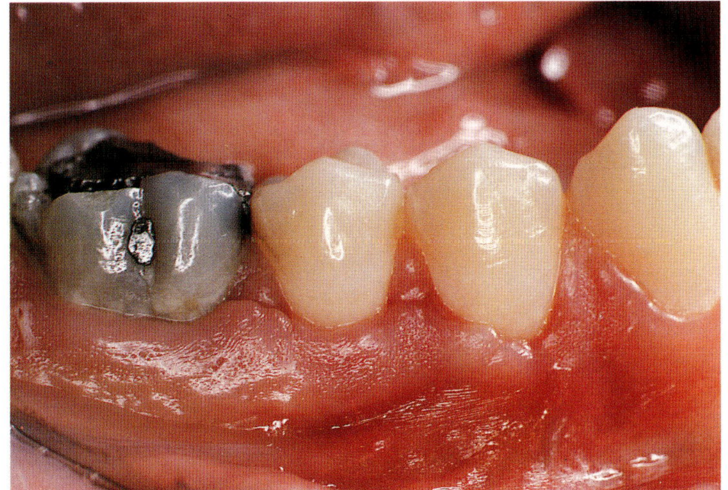

- One week followup:
  - monitor soft tissue healing
  - stress oral hygiene

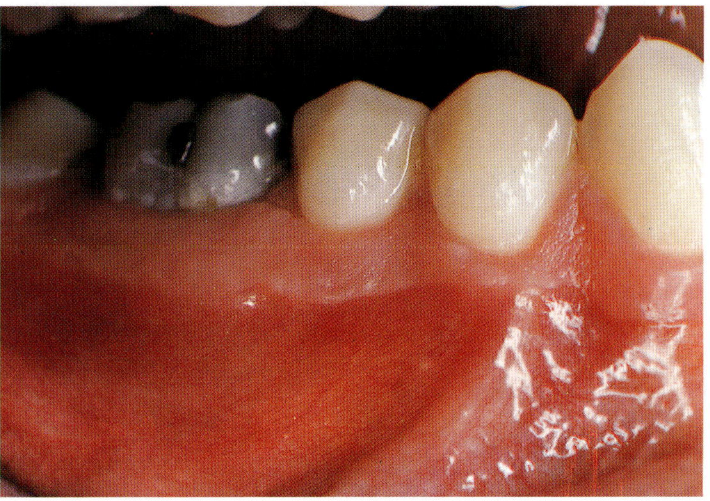

- One month followup:
  - tissues are firmly attached
  - asymptomatic and fully functional

11 Maxillary Molar Surgery

Endodontic surgery involving the maxillary first and second molars presents a unique set of circumstances not common to other regions of the oral cavity. Anatomic structures such as the maxillary sinus, malar process, palatal root, heavy buttressed bone, the morphologic configuration of the mesial-buccal roots, and the intimate juxtaposition of the maxillary sinus to these roots complicates the surgical approach.

Long roots or a malar process that dips more inferiorly than usual can create a thick bony housing over the mesial-buccal root, which makes locating the apex difficult. Often, the mesial-buccal root has a prominent eminence in its entire length. This usually facilitates apex location when the apical third of the root is used as a guide. The cortical bone in the molar region demands accurate endometrics, especially if the guiding eminence is not present. Beneath the cortical plate is the vascular medullary bone, which can be a source of bleeding, making visibility difficult.

The relationship of the mesial-buccal root of the maxillary molar to the maxillary sinus is an important consideration. This close relationship, however, is not a contraindication when considering apical surgery in this region. Serious complications from sinus exposures are rare. Proper surgical techniques and primary closure reduce the possibility of sinus contamination. Patients should always be informed that there is a likelihood the sinus may be intruded on; however, they should also be assured that such an occurrence can easily be dealt with.

Elective endodontic surgery on maxillary molars of patients with acute sinusitis should be deferred. Ostia blockage prevents drainage, thus changing the sinus environment and facilitating the growth of anaerobic organisms. Surgery under these conditions could compound an already existing problem.

The presence of a second canal or an oblong isthmus in the mesiobuccal root of maxillary molars must always be anticipated. Without good visibility, such details can be missed. The use of the fiberoptic light source and optical magnification plays an important role in detecting these morphologic variations. Mesial-buccal roots also tend to be inclined distally and somewhat medially.

Because there are significant differences to the surgical approach to palatal roots, chapter 12 deals with them in more detail.

Surgical technique notes

Flap design

A full mucoperiosteal triangular flap offers excellent visibility. A rectangular flap can be used, but additional suturing is required and visibility in the posterior vestibule is difficult. The Ochsenbein-Luebke flap, although not ideal, can be used, but a thick band of attached marginal gingiva and high muscle attachments should dictate its use.

Incision

Place the vertical incision one to two teeth anterior to the tooth in question. Avoid any eminence or muscle attachments. A small, angled, releasing incision distal to the second molar may also be placed to facilitate reflection and prevent tearing of the flap.

Intrasulcular incisions follow tooth contours, dipping interproximally to free the marginal gingiva and papilla.

Flap reflection

Use a no. 4 Molt curet beginning at the midportion of the vertical incision, reflecting against a quartered gauze held under light pressure. The presence of buttressed bone during reflection can cause slippage and perforation.

Flap retraction

Either a no. 23 Seldin or a Minnesota retractor with a fiberoptic attachment can be used. Either retractor directs an excellent point light source on the surgical field. Because tissue is firmly attached in the malar region, facial bruising can result from pressure exerted during flap retraction.

Cortical bone exploration

Explore the surface of the cortical bone with an endodontic explorer to identify bony defects. Use physiological or pathologic fenestrations as guides for osseous access.

Osseous access

Using the bony contour of the mesial-buccal root in the apical third, remove cortical bone over the root. After identifying the root surface, direct the removal apically until the apex is visualized and defined.

Root end exposure

Enlarge the bony access in the apical area. Ensure that the entire apex is seen and defined on its lateral boundaries. If a lesion exists, free the boundaries mesially, distally, superiorly, and along the root surface. *Do not thrust into the lesion medially* or intrusion into the maxillary sinus wall may occur. If at this point the lesion cannot be enucleated, the root may have to be resected first. Careless use of the curet into and around the lesion increases the chances of sinus invasion.

Root resection

Resect the root with a fissure bur at a 45-degree angle. Initially, the bur should rest laterally on the root surface extending the entire buccal-lingual dimension of the root. Then resect laterally with an unimpeded sweeping motion. *Do not direct the bur medially during the resection—only laterally;* this will protect against perforation of the sinus.

Root end inspection

The cut root end is inspected via fiberoptics and visual magnification. Observe for the second canal or any unfilled isthmuses that may be present. At this time the lesion may be removed, if present. If the sinus is suspected to have been intruded upon, ask the patient to hold his or her nose and blow gently. The membrane will show movement or there will be an escape of air and bubbles, which are easily noted. When a lesion is attached to the mucosa of the sinus, remove what is possible from solid bone and leave the remainder. Any tissue removed should be submitted for biopsy. *Do not attempt cureting into the sinus to remove tissue that cannot be seen, defined, or clearly identified.* Before irrigating, carefully pack *Nu Gauze* on the sinus wall *but not into the sinus.* Irrigate gently with saline *and without intense pressure.* Do not use the airblown water syringe or a handpiece, which may blow water and air into the sinus.

Root end preparation

Use a Class I preparation if a single canal is present. Use a slot preparation if two canals and an isthmus are present. The microhandpiece is ideally suited for this procedure. Carefully pack the osseous defect with *Nu Gauze* and dry the apical preparation with the cut end of paper points held in a cotton pliers.

Retrograde obturation

Place the retrograde obturation material of choice and remove excess debris with copious irrigation and suction. Remove the *Nu Gauze* packing and irrigate the entire surgical site. Take a confirmation radiograph before final closure.

Final closure

The repositioning and readaptation of the flap, as well as the fibrin clot, create an excellent barrier if an intrusion into the maxillary sinus occurred. The suturing should be snug but not tight, creating complete closure and avoiding tissue tears. If there has been a suspected intrusion into the sinus, the patient is instructed to limit blowing the nose and to sneeze with the mouth open. A drinking straw should not be used for the next 5 days. Antibiotics and decongestants, although not indicated at this point in therapy, have been by convention prescribed. Based on the clinician's clinical experience and the patient's medical history, prophylactic antibiotics and decongestants may be a part of therapy. Some patients experience a slight oozing from the nose, but this is usually short lived and of little consequence. Analgesics are prescribed accordingly. The patient is appointed for suture removal if the sutures are not absorbable, and healing is monitored on a normal followup basis.

Presurgical Radiographic Examination

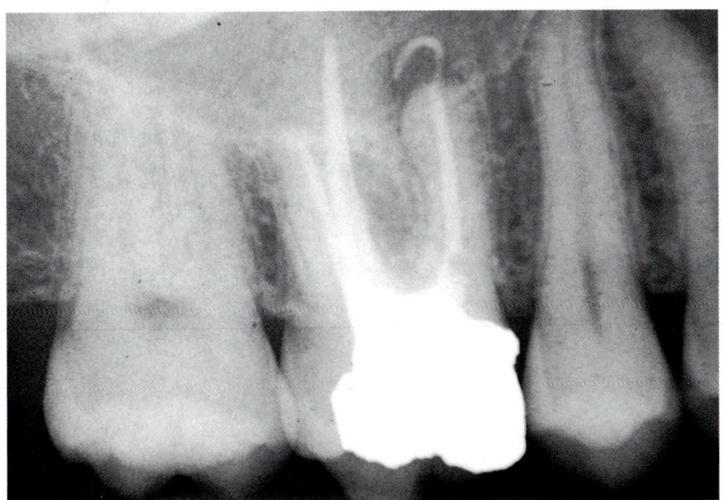

- Review for:
  - previous root canal treatment
  - overextension of mesial-buccal root
  - periapical radiolucency on mesial-buccal root
  - proximity of maxillary sinus

Presurgical Soft Tissue Examination

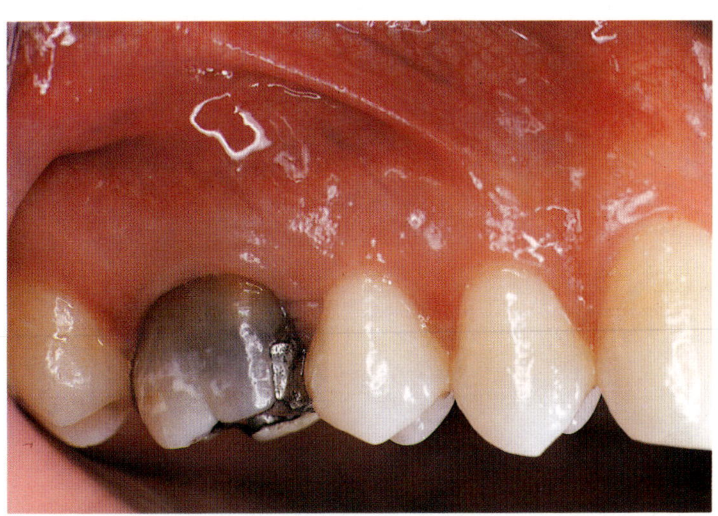

- Evaluate for:
  - muscle attachments
  - vestibular depth
  - attached gingiva
  - gingival health

Anatomic Landmarks

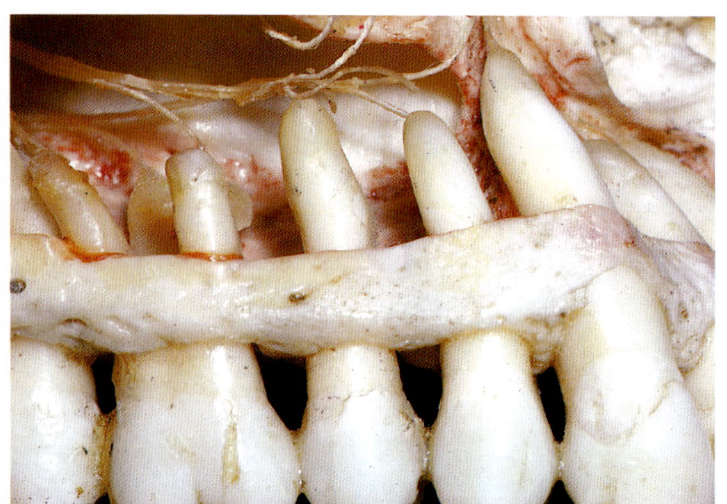

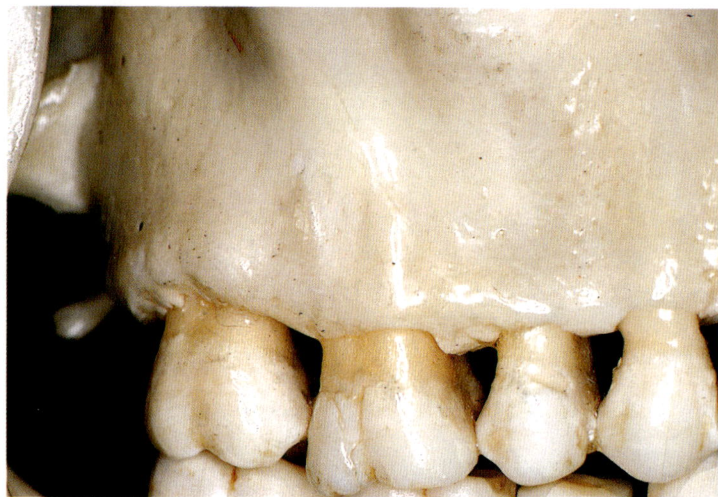

- Maxillary sinus.
- Malar process.
- Buttressed bone.
- Root eminences.
- Thickness of cortical bone.

Flap Design

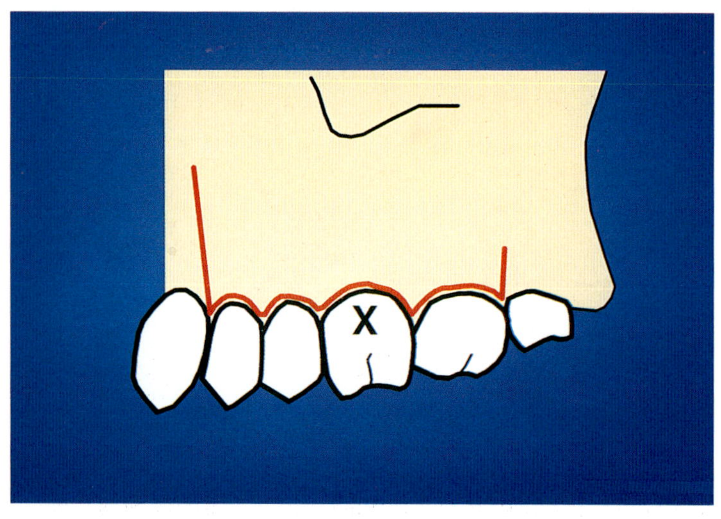

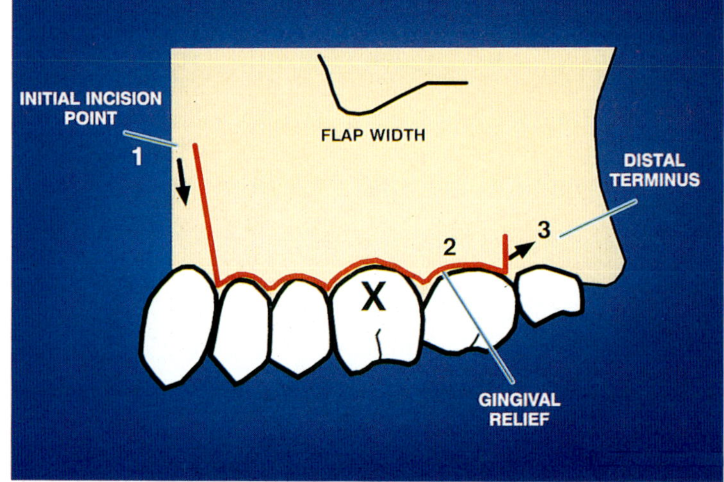

- Triangular flap with distal relaxing incision:
  - initial incision point
  - gingival relief
  - distal terminus

Incision

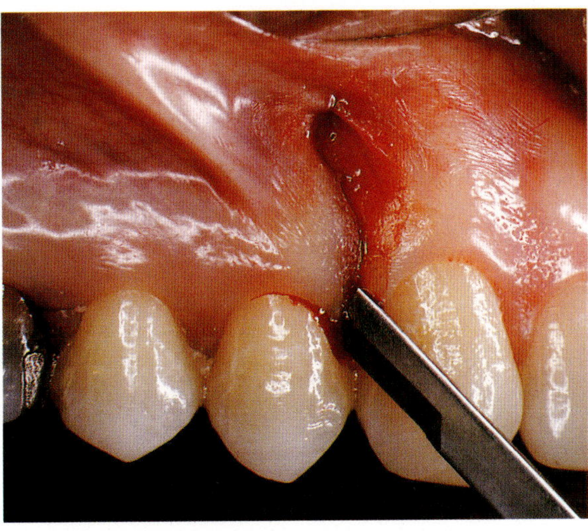

- Vertical incision:
  - —anterior to muscle attachments
  - —avoid eminences
  - —through periosteum to bone

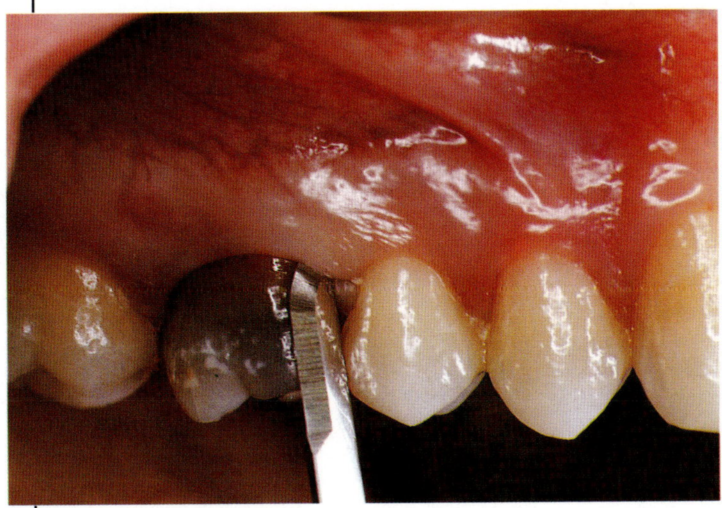

- Horizontal incision:
  - —intrasulcular
  - —follows contours of crowns
  - —incise to depth of crestal bone

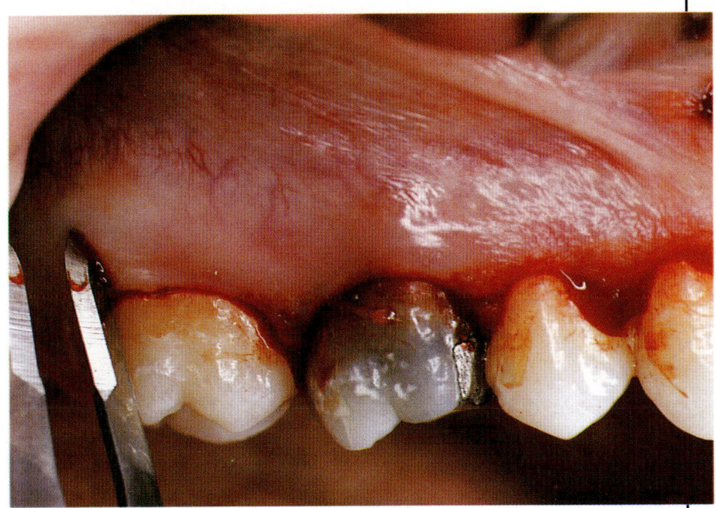

- Distal releasing incision:
  - —distal to second molar
  - —prevents stretching and tearing of flap
  - —allows unimpeded reflection

Flap Reflection

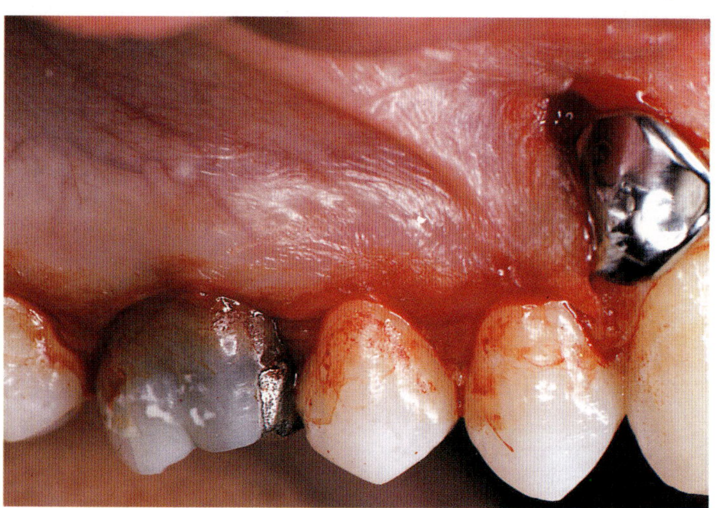

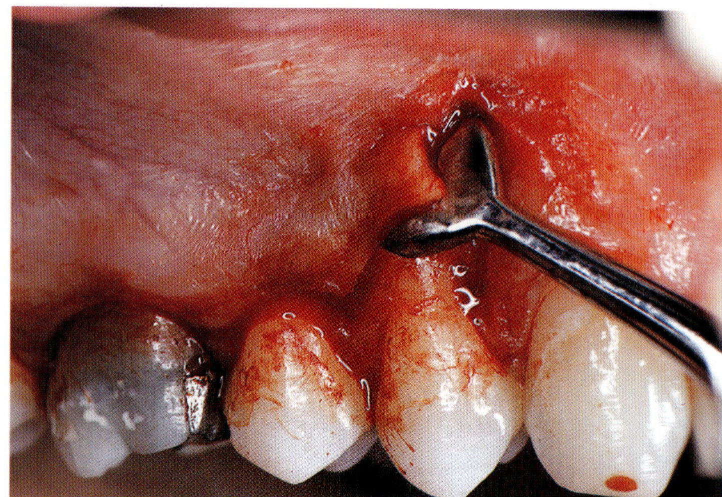

- No. 4 Molt curet.
- Initiate at midportion — vertical incision.
- Undermining elevation.
- Direct reflection posteriorly and superiorly.
- Buttressed bone can impede reflection.

Flap Retraction

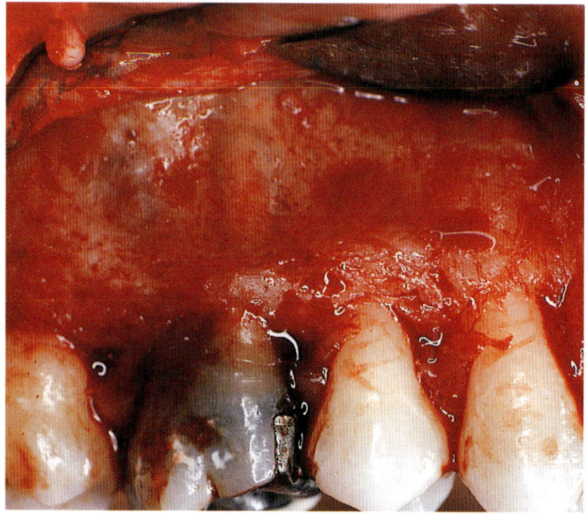

- Fiberoptic retractors:
  - — no. 23 Seldin
  - — Minnesota
- Retractor placement:
  - — perpendicular to bone
  - — free of soft tissue impingement

Exploration of Cortical Plate

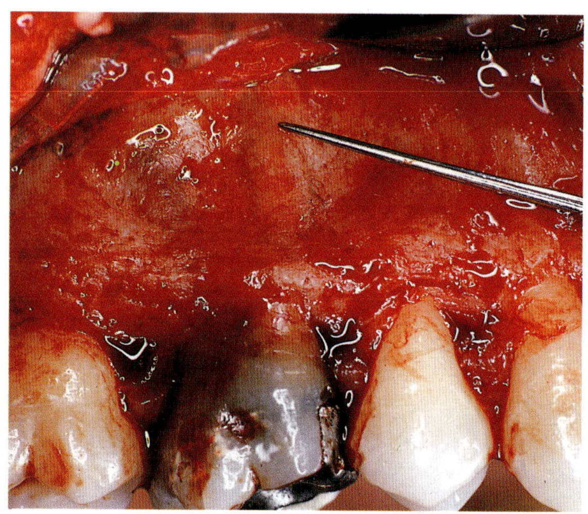

- Probe surface.
- Identify defects:
  - — pathologic
  - — physiologic
- Identify apical third root contour.

Initial Bone Removal

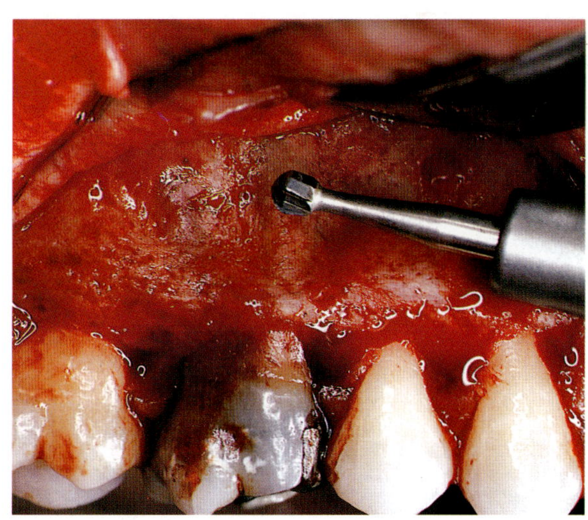

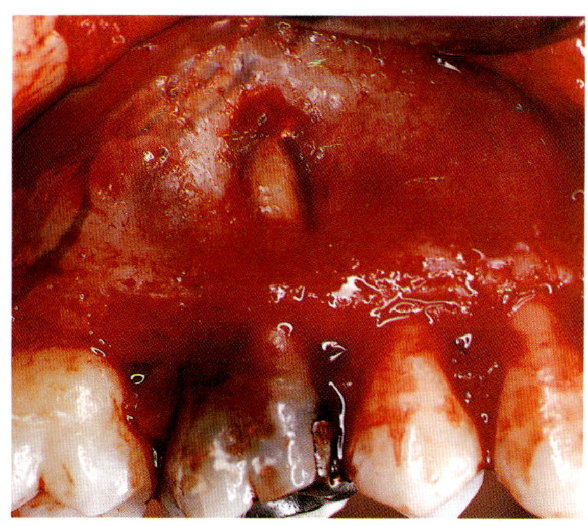

- Use root contour.
- Begin at apical third.
- Penetrate bone to root surface.
- Use root as guide to apex.

Osseous Access Completed

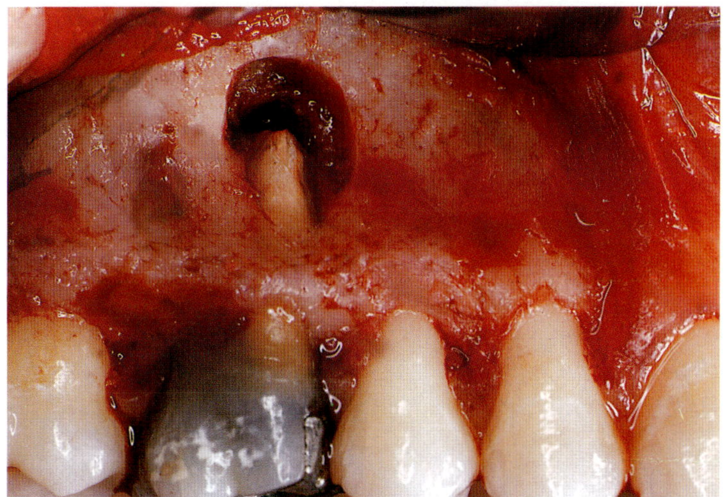

- Lesion/foreign body removed.
- Limits of apex defined.
- Root end beveled and inspected.

Resected Mesial-Buccal Root

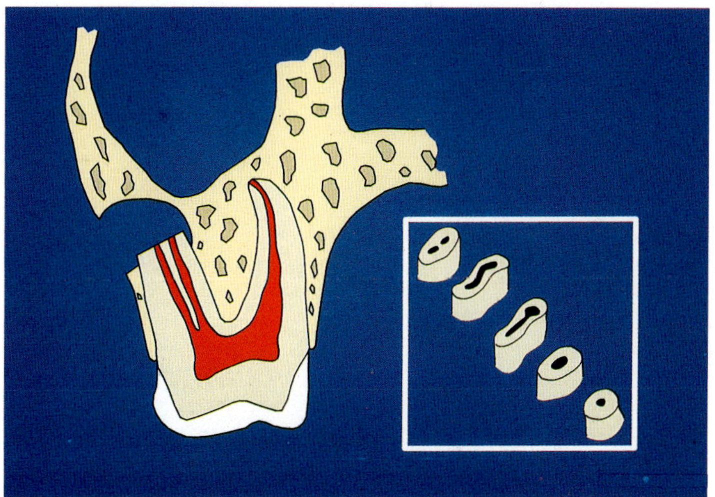

- Angled for visualization.
- Multiple canal configurations.
- Note position within bony housing and relationship to the maxillary sinus.

Radiographic Confirmation

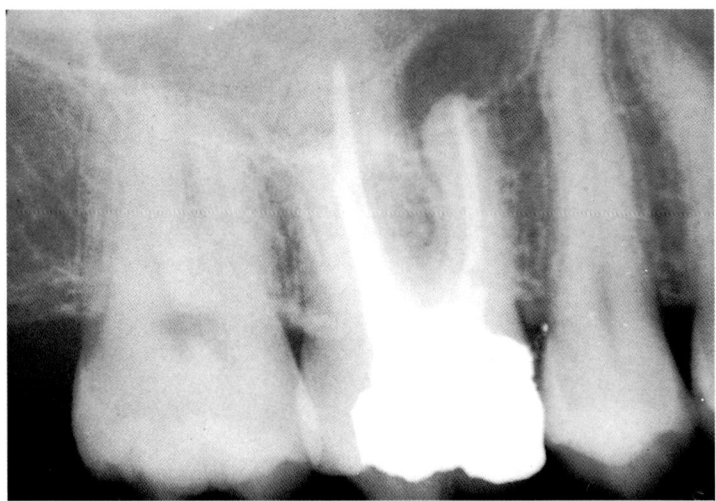

- Take radiograph before closure.
- Inspect for apical debris/foreign material.

12 Maxillary Molar Palatal Root Surgery

Endodontic surgery on palatal roots of maxillary molars has not been discussed at length in the dental literature. However, conditions can present where this type of surgical procedure must be considered. In the past, contraindications to performing this surgery included poor visibility, inadequate access to the surgical site, the proximity of the greater palatine artery, and the location of the maxillary sinus. However, all of these previous contraindications are easily dealt with by applying basic sound surgical principles and current technologies.

Although the concern always exists that the greater palatine artery can be encroached upon during surgery, familiarity with palatal anatomy and the use of sound surgical technique reduce the possibility of this occurrence and make the procedure clinically feasible. The greater palatine artery exits from the greater palatine canal. The canal is situated lingual to the maxillary second molar, between the inner plate of the alveolar process and the midline of the palate. The neurovascular bundle runs anteriorly, usually in a groove or depression, which gives it added protection. Careful evaluation and flap design will prevent encroachment on the palatine artery.

Surgical technique notes

Presurgical preparation

A full maxillary arch alginate impression is taken as the first step in preparing a maxillary stent. The stent serves as a support for the flap and facilitates repositioning and readaptation as well as hemorrhage control. Hemostasis is enhanced by pressure from the stent and is essential for healing, especially in the event of an encroachment on the palatal artery.

Two casts are poured and trimmed. The first cast is used to fabricate a *clear acrylic resin stent.* Alternatively, a stent can be made from the clear soft mouthguard material and vacuum formed for an exact adaptation. It is used by many clinicians because of its simplicity, flexibility, added retention, and ease of removal and placement.

After the stent is removed from the model, it is trimmed and any irregularities are eliminated. The stent must always be tried in before surgery. Pressure points are relieved as is any excessive palatal extension. The second cast is trimmed in cross-section starting distally and moving anteriorly until the entire distal surface of the maxillary first molar is outlined. The cross-sectional model reveals the vertical and horizontal dimensions of the palatal vault. This information is useful in estimating the proximity of the palatal root in relationship to the palatal cortical plate.

Flap design

Use a modified envelope flap with a *small* vertical relaxing incision (2 to 4 mm) at the distal lingual line angle of the maxillary second molar. The horizontal component is an intrasulcular incision that uses the lingual contours of the posterior and anterior teeth as a guide. Buttressed bone is frequently encountered, and care must be exercised to keep the incision on bone. The palatal gingiva is very thick and fibrous and the incision must free the marginal gingiva prior to reflection.

Flap reflection and retraction

The palatal tissue is characteristically thick and fibrous and requires effort in reflection and retraction. It is sometimes very firmly attached to the irregular and heavily textured bone of the posterior palate. A palatal suture tie is an important adjunct in facilitating tissue retraction and enhancing the visual field of the surgical site. The suture tie is easily secured interproximally on the opposite side. Because of the limited access and visibility at the surgical site, the use of a fiberoptic light source on a no. 23 Seldin retractor delivers a point source of light directly onto the surgical defect and surrounding bony surface, enhancing visibility.

Cortical bone exploration

When dealing with palatal root surgery the most common finding is a pathologic fenestration on the palatal cortical plate. On occasion, perforations of the root and overextended gutta percha points as well as large apical lesions can be observed.

Osseous access

As mentioned earlier, the cross-sectional cast shows variations in palatal vault height and width. Palates that have narrow (high) vaults usually have a palatal root that is closer to the palatal cortical bone. Vaults that are wide (low) usually have a palatal root that is further away from the palatal cortical bone. If a large periapical lesion and pathologic fenestration are not present, the surgical access window will have to be prepared through thick cortical bone and widened sufficiently so the entire apical root third can be visualized. Failure to accomplish this will result in poor visualization of the surgical site and is a major contributor to incomplete root resection.

Root end exposure

In most cases there is a buccal curvature of the apical third of the palatal root. Visual confirmation of both apical and lateral boundaries of this root are required before resection. The maxillary sinus, for the most part, is superior and lateral to the palatal root. It may dip down closer to the alveolar ridge where there is an edentulous area.

Root end resection

After complete visualization of the root apex and lateral boundaries is obtained, the root is ready for resection. *Never resect a root that is not clearly defined.* Place a fissure bur laterally on the root surface, angled at about 45 degrees, and make the cut in a mesial to distal direction in a continuous motion. Avoid any unnecessary superior and lateral thrusts of the bur, and remain on the clearly defined lateral root surface. The oval surface of this broad root will be clearly and easily defined.

Root end preparation and retrograde obturation

A Class I amalgam preparation is prepared with the microhandpiece. The surgical defect can be packed with *Nu Gauze* for hemorrhage control. The amalgam is placed with the microcarrier and condensed with the modified no. 23 explorer cut to size. Excess amalgam can be removed with irrigation and suction; the *Nu Gauze* should be removed at this time.

Final closure

Take a confirmation radiograph before final closure and suturing. Irrigate beneath the flap to remove any packed debris that has gone unnoticed. Then readapt and reposition the tissue and place the stent. Keep the stent in place for about 5 minutes to facilitate readaptation and repositioning of the palatal tissue; this prevents pooling of tissue fluids and blood. Carefully remove the stent and place a single suspensory suture around the involved tooth. Complete the final suturing with single interrupted interproximal sutures. Replace the stent and dismiss the patient until the next day for stent removal and observation. The stent is not usually kept *in place* for more than 1 day. If you decide to keep the stent in place for an extra day, remove and irrigate it with sterile saline.

Followup

After the stent is removed, healing is monitored. Sutures are removed in 3 to 5 days and the patient placed on followup.

Presurgical Radiographic Examination

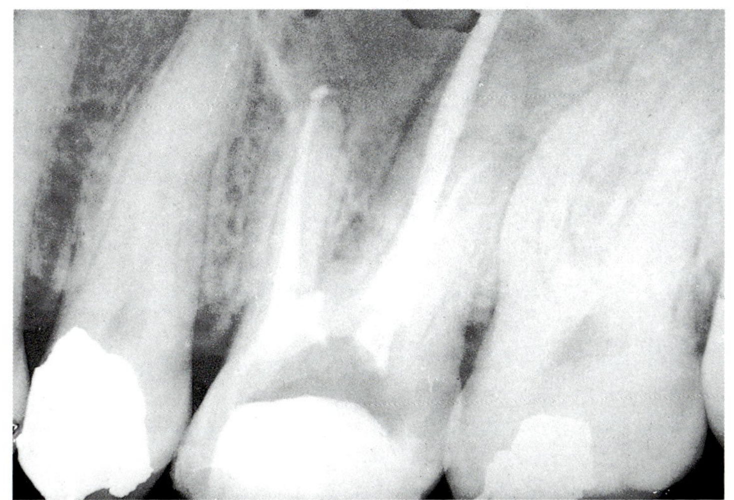

- Review for:
  - overextended palatal obturation/perforation
  - root length
  - maxillary sinus

Presurgical Soft Tissue Examination

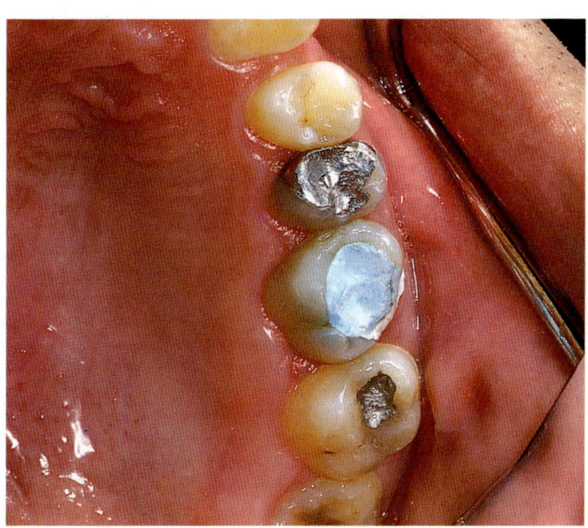

- Findings:
  - intact, noninflamed periodontium
  - no swelling or sinus tract
  - high palatal vault

Palatal Landmarks

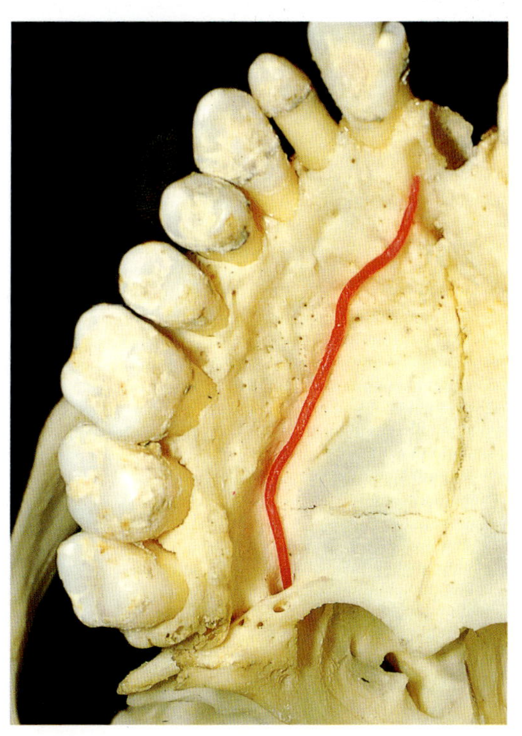

- Greater palatine foramen.
- Alveolar-palatal junction.
- Path of neurovascular bundle.

High Palatal Vault

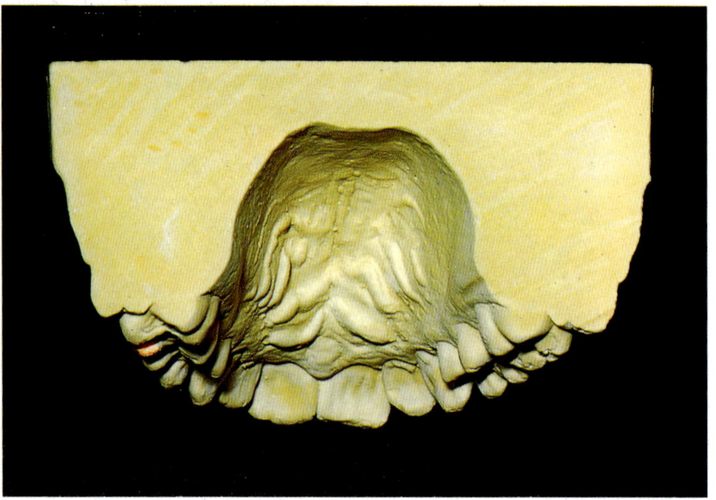

- Thin cortical bone.
- Favorable access.
- Root end proximity closer to cortical bone.

Shallow Palatal Vault

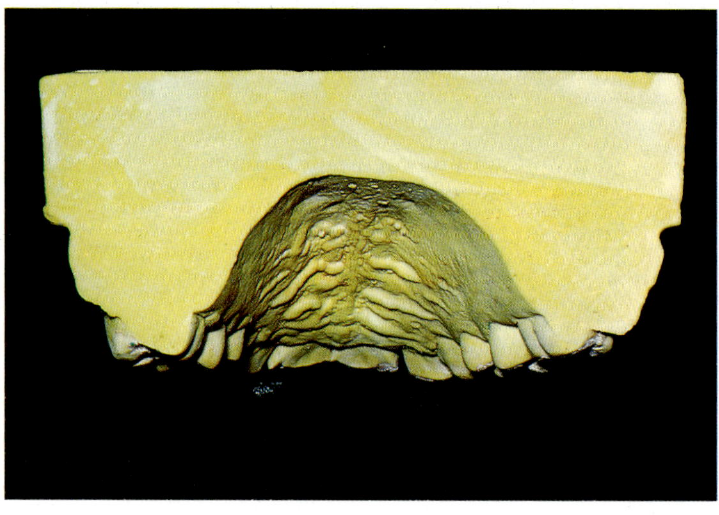

- Thick cortical bone.
- Limited access.
- Absence of root eminences.
- Root end more distant from cortical bone.

Palatal Root Configuration Within High and Low Vault Housing

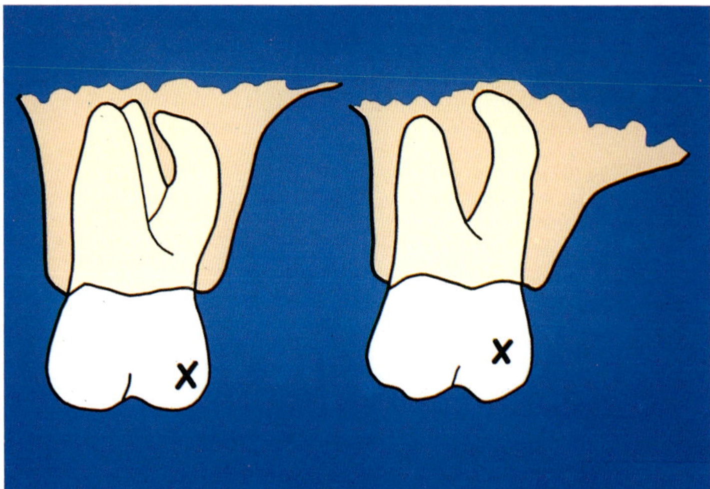

- Root anatomy:
  - —buccal curvature of palatal root
  - —length of palatal root
  - —oval cross-sectional configuration
  - —convex palatal surface
  - —concave furcal surface

Acrylic Resin Palatal Support

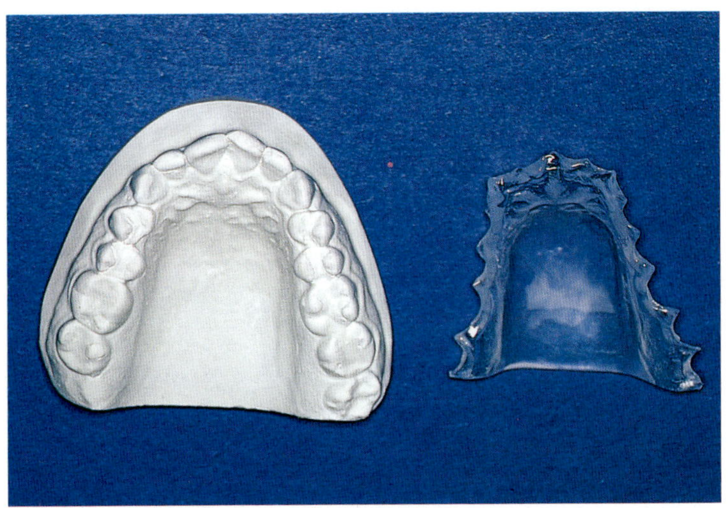

- Study model taken before surgery.
- Clear acrylic resin stent.

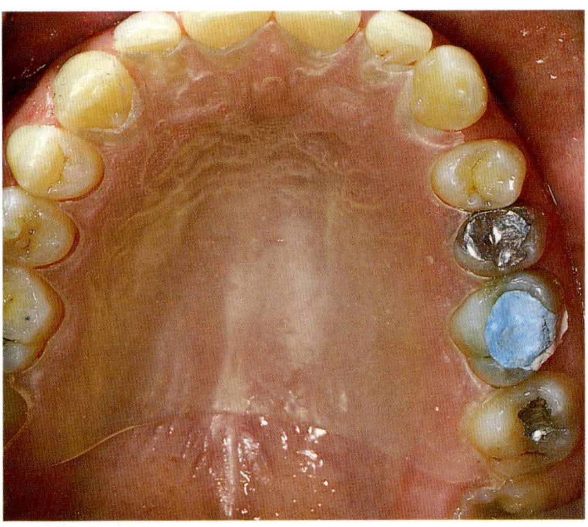

- Presurgical try-in.
- Adjust pressure points and palatal extension.
- Stent facilitates:
  - flap repositioning
  - flap support
  - hemorrhage control

Palatal Flap Design

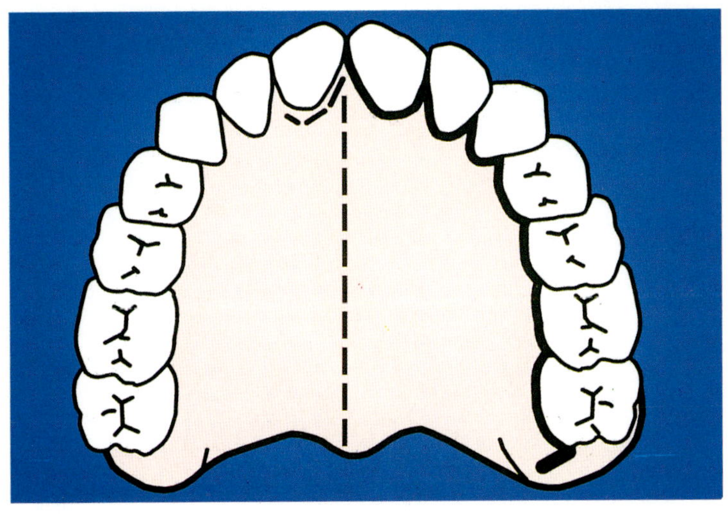

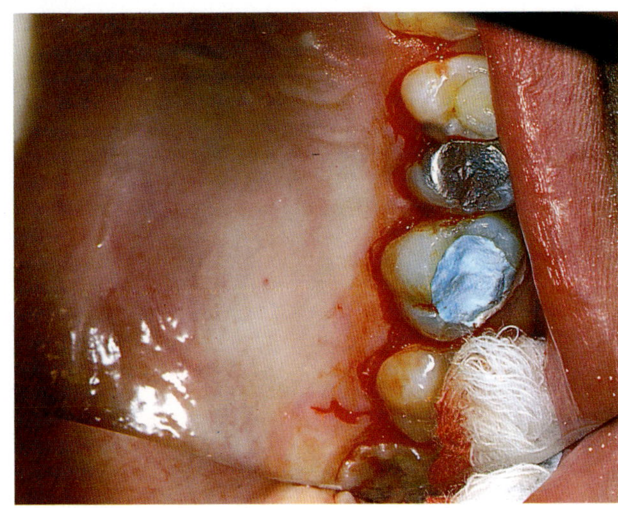

- Modified envelope flap:
  - intrasulcular incision extending to the central incisor
  - vertical releasing incision (2 to 4 mm) at the distal-lingual line angle of the second molar

Flap Reflection

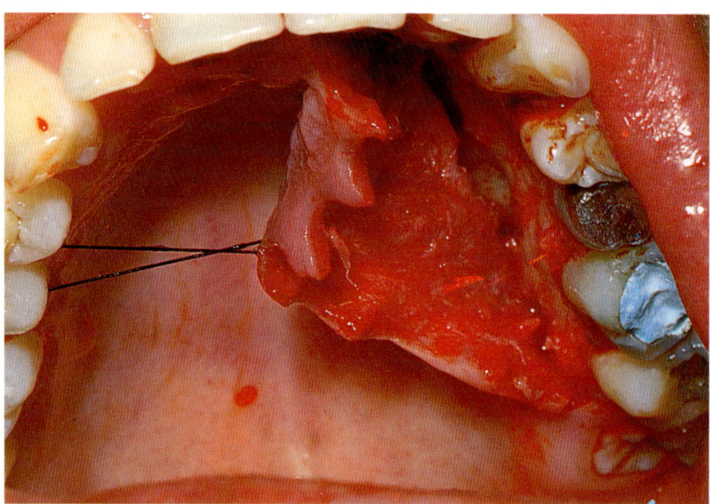

- Distal vertical relaxing incision with anterior envelope design.
- Thick, fibrous palatal mucosa.
- Irregularly textured palatal bone.
- Suture tied from flap to opposite arch:
  - facilitates retraction
  - enhances visibility

Flap Retraction/Osseous Access

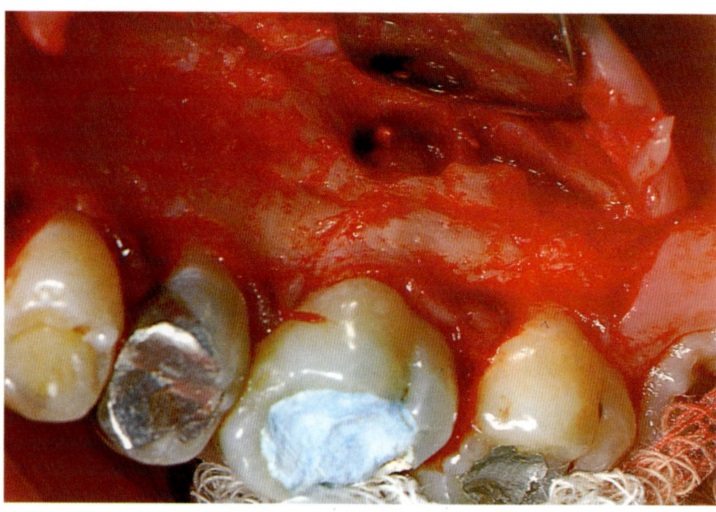

- No. 23 Seldin retractor with fiberoptic attachment.
- Check for pathologic fenestration.
- Maintain retractor on bone.
- Establish osseous access.
- Isolate root apex.
- Inspect root end and treat according to findings:
  - apical curettage
  - apical resection
  - apical resection with retrograde obturation

Palatal Root Anomalies

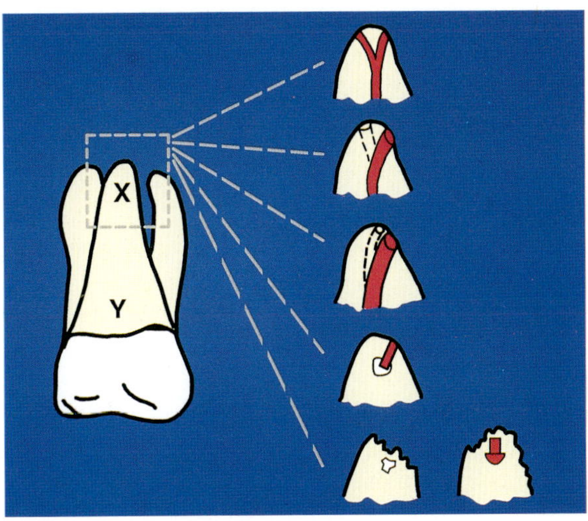

- Canal delta configuration.
- Foramen transport.
- Root perforation.
- Overextension.
- Root resorption.

Clinical Perforation/Overextension

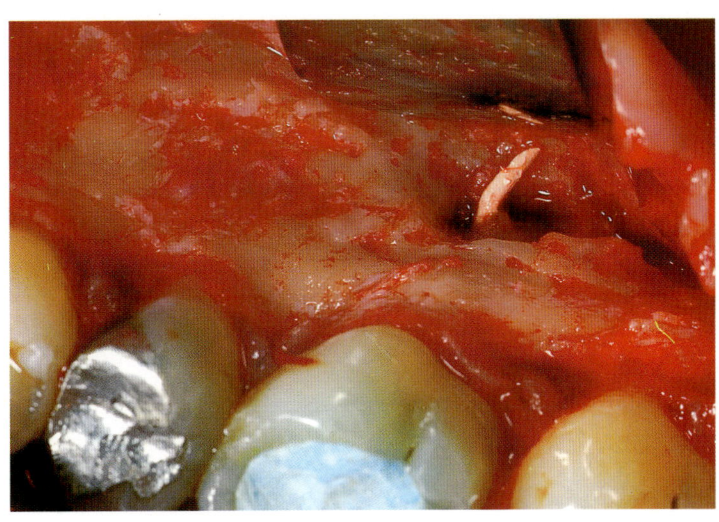

- Tissue reflected.
- Pathologic bone fenestration.
- Overextended gutta-percha point visible after removal of pathologic tissue.

Root Resection

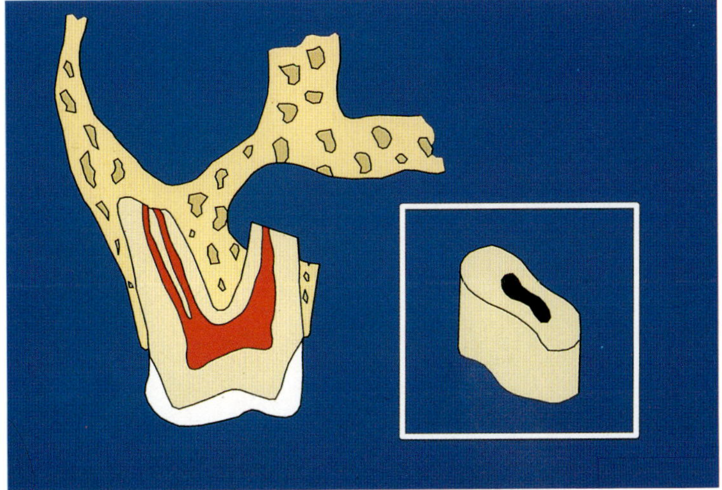

- Angled for visualization.
- Note position within bony housing and relationship to the maxillary sinus.

Retrograde Preparation and Obturation

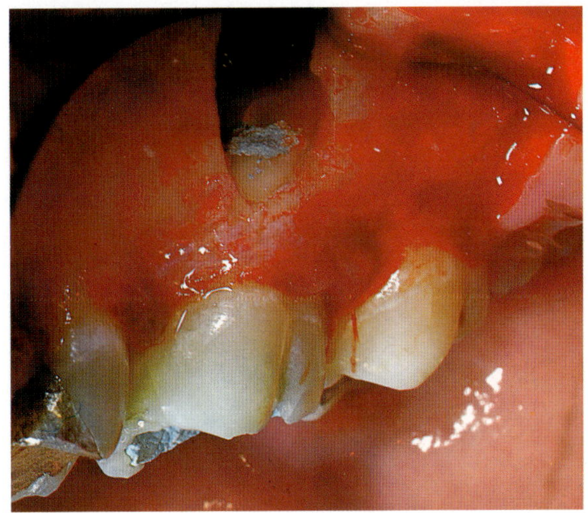

- Use microhead handpiece.
- Place hemorrhage control packing.
- Class I amalgam retrograde obturation.

Radiographic Confirmation

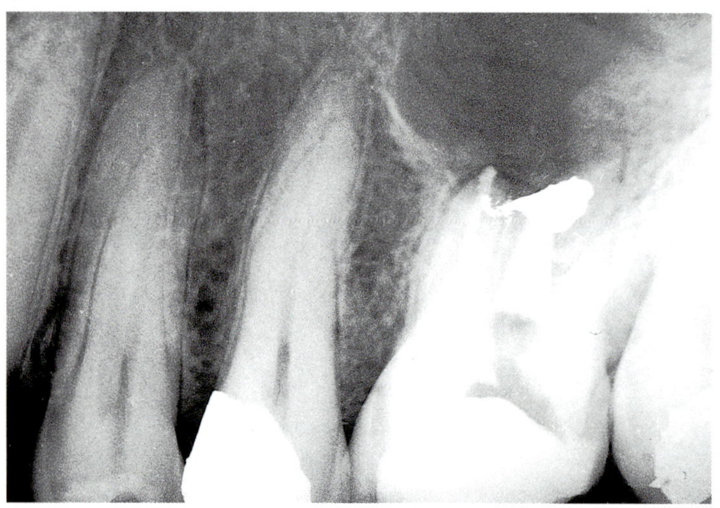

- Take radiograph before closure.
- Detect foreign debris.
- Confirm complete resection.
- Remove hemorrhage control packing.

Palatal Stent Placement

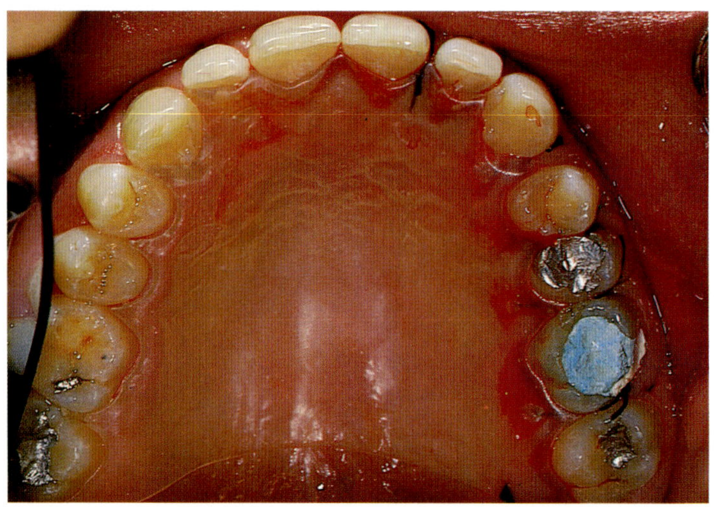

- Place temporarily (for 5 minutes):
  - facilitates flap repositioning
  - eliminates pooled blood
  - establishes initial attachment and clotting
- Place after suturing:
  - facilitates flap support
  - prevents hematoma formation

Postsurgical Followup

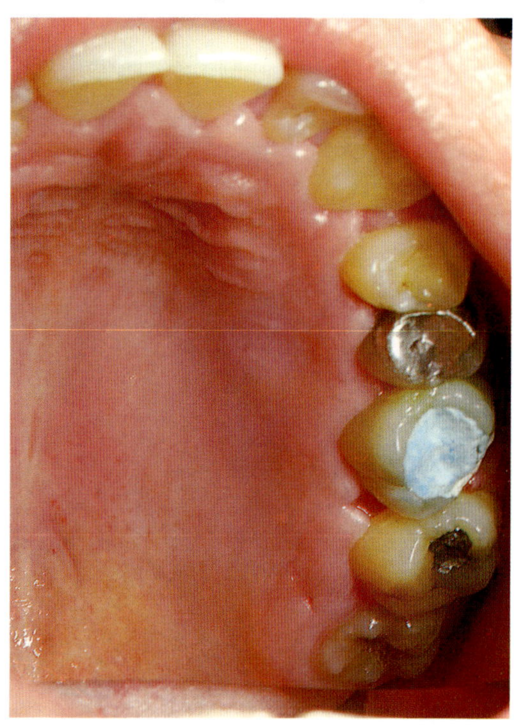

- Remove stent the day after surgery.
- Remove sutures after 3 to 5 days.
- Schedule regular followup appointment to monitor healing.

13 Postsurgical Complications

Throughout this atlas, basic surgical principles have been discussed at length. The intent has been to demonstrate that if these guidelines are followed, the incidence of postsurgical complications could be significantly reduced.

However, despite care and concern on the part of the surgeon, postsurgical problems can occur. The clinician must be quick to recognize them and must understand their etiology and methods of treatment.

Postsurgical technique notes

Pain

Aspirin-containing compounds should be discontinued before a surgical procedure and as a rule not prescribed as an analgesic after the completion of surgery. Nonsteroidal antiinflammatory drugs (NSAIDS) are excellent substitutes for aspirin. A helpful hint in coping with postsurgical pain is to preoperatively dose the patient with an NSAID of choice (eg, ibuprofen 400 mg 1 hour before surgery). NSAIDS appear to be more than sufficient for mild to moderate pain. A stronger analgesic level is required in cases where severe pain is anticipated or patient tolerance indicates such; the prescribing of a narcotic may be indicated. In general, severe pain and discomfort from endodontic surgical procedures has not been a major problem. Patients appear to tolerate these procedures well.

Swelling

Swelling is an expected sequela from endodontic surgery. It can range from minimal to moderate and, in rare cases, severe. The incidence of postsurgical swelling can be reduced when sound surgical techniques are followed. Included in these techniques are: incisions that do not penetrate muscle, complete reflection of the periosteum, placement of the retractor on bone, and proper readaptation of the flap. The application of ice and pressure to the affected side will also reduce postsurgical swelling. Rarely is swelling the result of frank infection.

Infection

Although an uncommon occurrence as a result of endodontic surgery, infection is nevertheless possible. When it occurs there is usually an underlying cause that has been overlooked. Avoid surgical procedures in the presence of poor oral hygiene and/or untreated periodontal disease. Undetected root fractures or a missed unfilled canal can be a source of postoperative infection. Debris under a flap or a flap that fails to attach can be a contributing factor as well. Foreign debris left in the surgical site during retrograde preparation must always be considered. Usually the infection is localized to the surgical site. Whenever swelling and infection are present, a temperature baseline must be established and a regional description of the swelling noted. Treatment will depend on the type, location, and severity of the infection. In such cases incision, drainage, and antibiotic therapy must be instituted. Culturing should be accomplished when possible. Followup is essential and considered a part of therapy.

Bleeding

Bleeding is primarily the result of failing to completely reflect the mucoperiosteum. Incisions deep into the surrounding tissue and through muscle attachments also contribute to bleeding and tissue hematoma formation. Poor tissue repositioning and readaptation, as well as suturing that leaves tissue spaces, are responsible for much of the oozing seen postsurgically. Frequently, torn sutures or trauma caused by overzealous toothbrushing are also recognized as causative factors. In addition, patient noncompliance to proper postsurgical application of pressure can be considered a leading cause of pooling and oozing of blood. In these cases diagnosis and treatment are easily accomplished.

Discoloration

Facial discoloration, while not a common occurrence, does happen and is cosmetically detracting. Patients who are fair skinned seem most susceptible. Care during reflection and especially retraction can reduce the incidence of bruising and discoloration. Avoid retractor pressure on the lips and soft tissue, especially in the region of the malar process, canine eminence, and mental foramen. Firm suturing and knot security also play an important role. Discoloration, although esthetically unappealing, will dissipate in several days. Discoloration will undergo several color changes before final resolution. Informing the patient before surgery of this possibility will reduce patient anxiety if bruising occurs.

Intraoral hematoma

Intraoral hematoma can present in a dramatic fashion. It can be localized or involve the submucosa of the entire lip or cheek. It usually originates as the result of tissue compression during retraction while operating in a restricted area. It is often seen in the anterior maxillary and mandibular premolar region. Intraoral hematomas dissipate within days and are not of any serious consequence.

Poor oral hygiene

When this condition exists preoperatively, elective surgery must be deferred because it will compromise healing and can lead to infection. Poor oral hygiene is frequently seen postsurgically as a white film on the mucosa over the surgical site and as plaque attached to sutures. Patients are frequently concerned about brushing in this area after surgery. Postsurgical oral hygiene is facilitated by the use of soft, disposable toothbrushes and antiplaque rinses (described in chapter 1). They are effective, are very well accepted by patients, and have shown excellent results.

Tissue trauma

Commissure of the lip. This can result from continued stretching during the surgical procedure as well as from inadvertent mechanical trauma from the straight handpiece during bone removal and root resection. The commissure should be lubricated with an ointment and protected by a retractor during use of the straight handpiece. Placement of a mouth block may be useful..

Vermillion border of the lip. Traumatic injury in this region can result because of excessive retractor pressure, unguarded mechanical trauma from the straight handpiece, and on occasion a heated instrument when used to remove gutta percha from the resected root. It can be a painful and unesthetic injury and can be prevented by extra care and concern during surgery.

Tissue trauma to the flap

Torn sutures. Suturing over eminences and prominent anatomic contours can cause tissue tension, compromised blood supply, and incision breakdown, resulting in torn sutures. Sutures under excessive tension and placed too close to the incision line are an additional cause of torn and displaced sutures. Sutures are rarely torn by brushing, but they can be loosened as a result of poor knot security. The use of a soft, disposable, toothbrush decreases knot and suture loss secondary to brushing.

Tissue dehiscence. This can result from improper incision placement, sutures under tension, and incision and sutures placed on bony eminences.

Incomplete root resection

An unusual occurrence, but one common to the inexperienced clinician, is the partial resection and obturation of the apical third of a root that has not been properly isolated, inspected, and defined. As previously stated, *never resect a root or attempt a retrograde obturation unless the apical third of the root can be seen and defined.*

Malalignment of retrograde obturation material

Because visibility can sometimes be compromised and the root end poorly isolated and defined, malalignment of the apical preparation can result. Diversion and perforation from the main canal will result in inaccurate placement of the retrograde obturation material. Proper visibility and the use of a fiberoptic light source at the surgical site may help prevent this occurrence.

Foreign debris in the surgical site

When apical amalgam is seen in a surgical site it is the result of poor apical isolation or lack of apical isolation. During retrograde obturation, an apical surgical pack of either bone wax, *Nu Gauze, Gelfoam,* or *Surgicel* should be used as a barrier. The microamalgam carrier quantitates the amount of amalgam placed. Custom-made condensers then direct the exact amounts of amalgam to the prepared site. Overflow of amalgam onto the bone should never be scraped, burnished, or removed by a bur. A saline lavage with adequate suction will easily remove the excess material. The amalgam debris can stain the mucosa, producing an unesthetic amalgam tattoo.

Paresthesia

Surgical procedures in the region of the mental foramen

and in close proximity to the mandibular neurovascular bundle can cause paresthesia of the lower lip, chin, and corner of the mouth. Whenever a surgical procedure is planned in this region, this issue should be discussed with the patient. The paresthesia can last from days to months and rarely is a permanent condition. If a paresthesia occurs, the area should be outlined by pin prick detection and duly noted in the record. This regional diagrammatic outline can be used in subsequent followup visits to monitor healing and nerve regeneration.

Pain

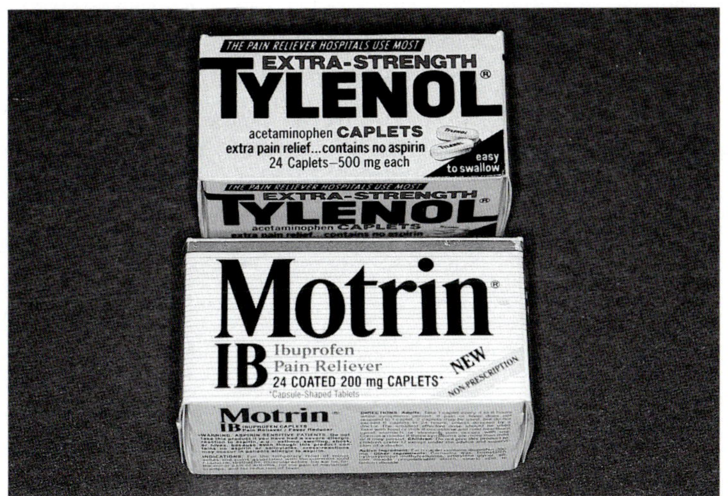

- Avoid aspirin-containing compounds.
- Medicate before surgery to reduce pain.
- Nonnarcotic medications:
  - use for mild to moderate pain
  - adequate for majority of cases
- Narcotic medications:
  - use for moderate to severe pain
  - not used routinely

Swelling

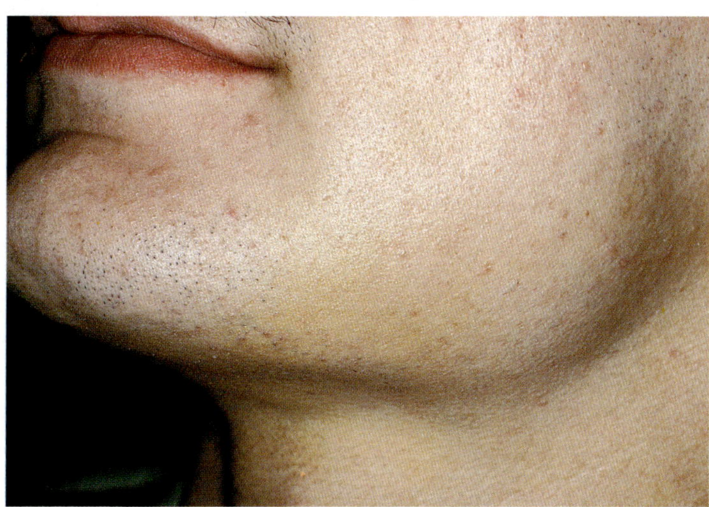

- Causes:
  - postsurgical edema
  - hematoma
  - infection

Infection

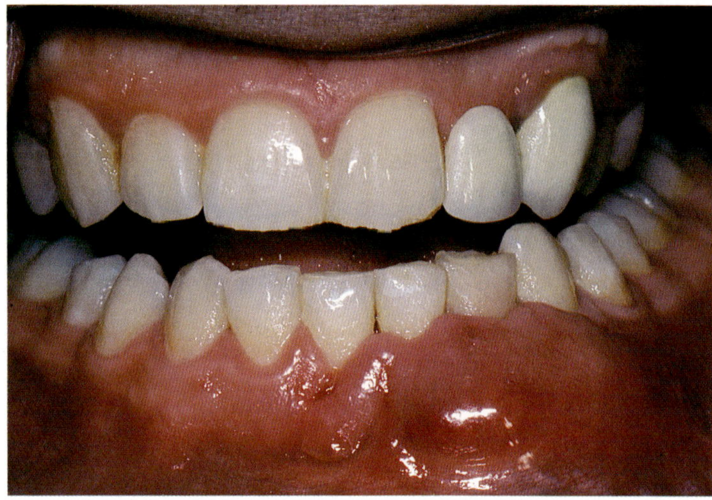

- Causes:
  - unfilled, infected canals
  - foreign debris in surgical site
  - fractured root
  - poor oral hygiene

Bleeding

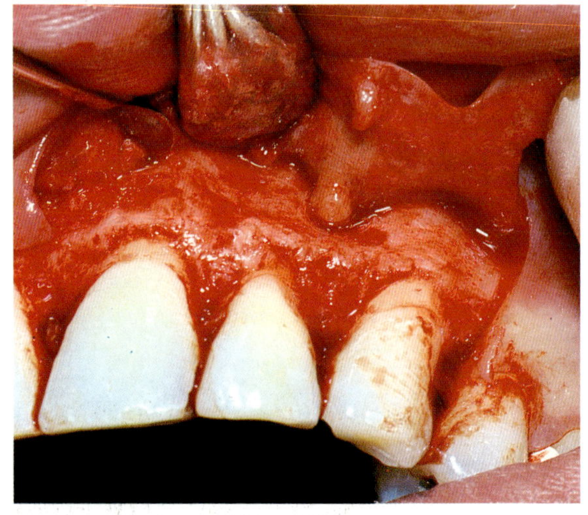

- Causes:
  - incomplete elevation of periosteum
  - incision into muscle attachments
  - impingement on flap during retraction

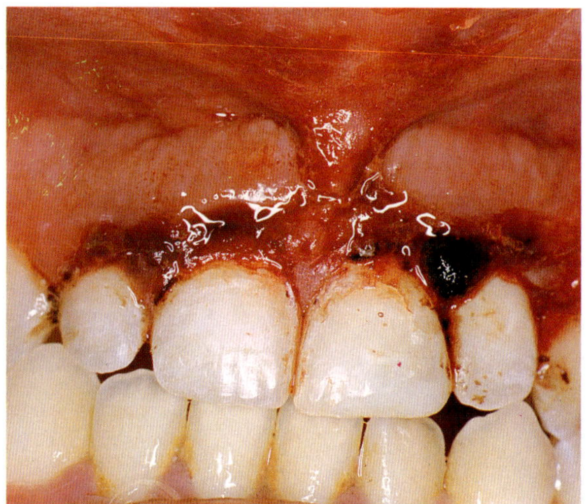

- Causes:
  - inadequate suturing
  - patient pulling on lip
  - toothbrush/mastication trauma postsurgery

Local Discoloration

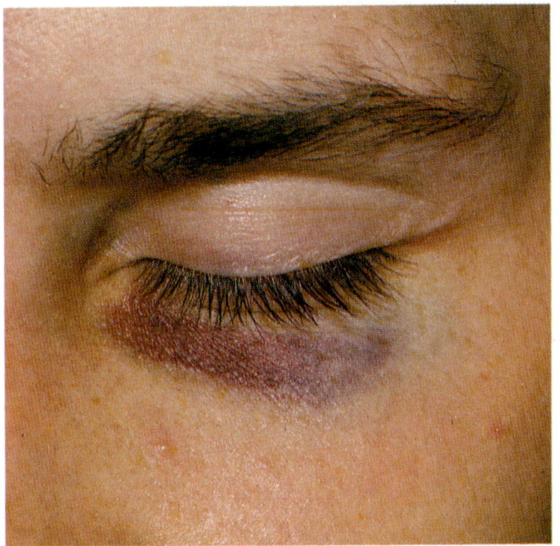

- Bruising.
- Compression of facial tissues secondary to intraoral reflection.
- Degree of discoloration is a function of:
  — site
  — complexion
  — degree of reflection trauma

General Discoloration

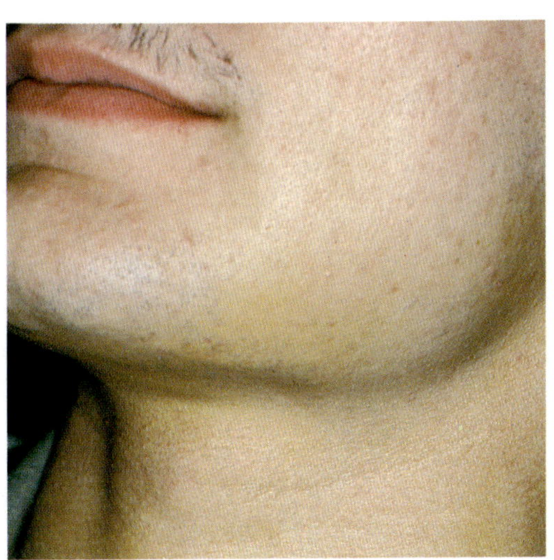

- External cutaneous.
- Diffuse hematoma with gravitational diffusion through fascial planes.

Intraoral Hematoma

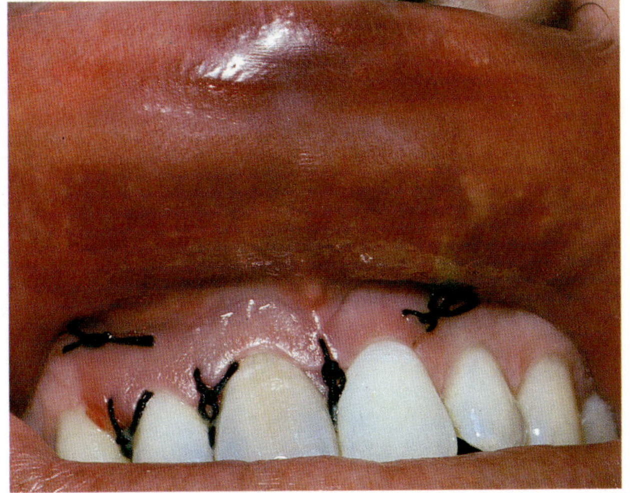

- Tissue compression during reflection.
- Failure to maintain retractor on bone.

Poor Oral Hygiene

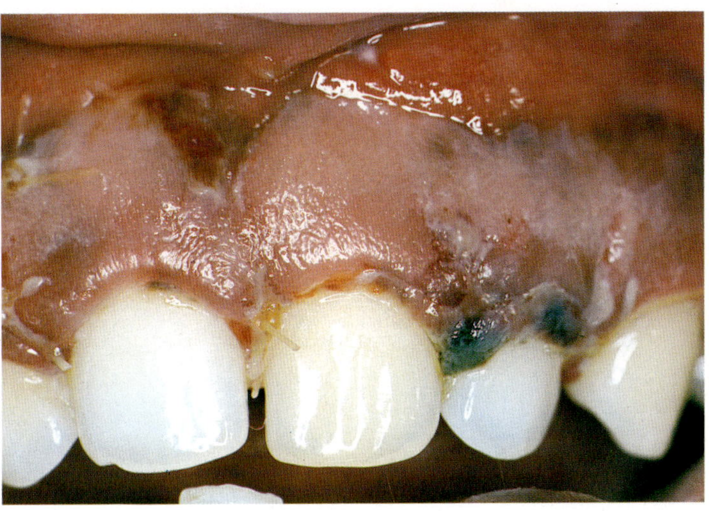

- Accumulata around teeth and sutures:
  — source of gingival inflammation
  — delays healing

Tissue Trauma

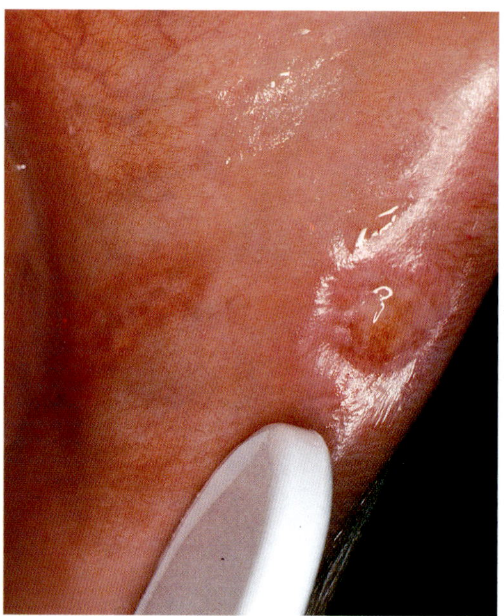

Cheek

- Inadequate bur protection.
- Inadequate tissue reflection.

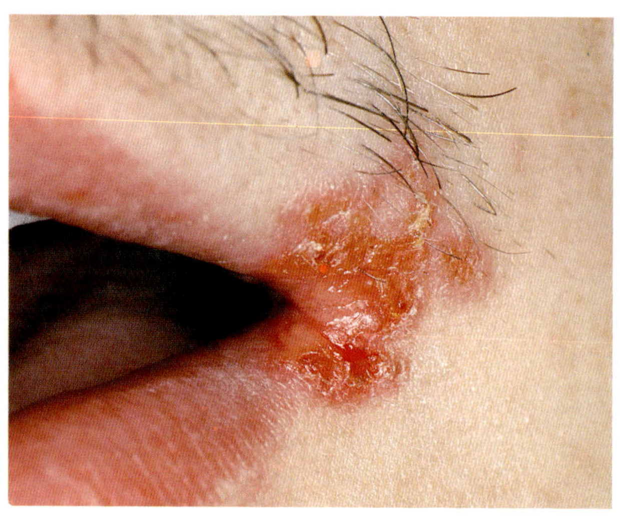

Commissure

- Limited oral access.
- Extensive stretching and manipulation.
- Inadequate lubrication.

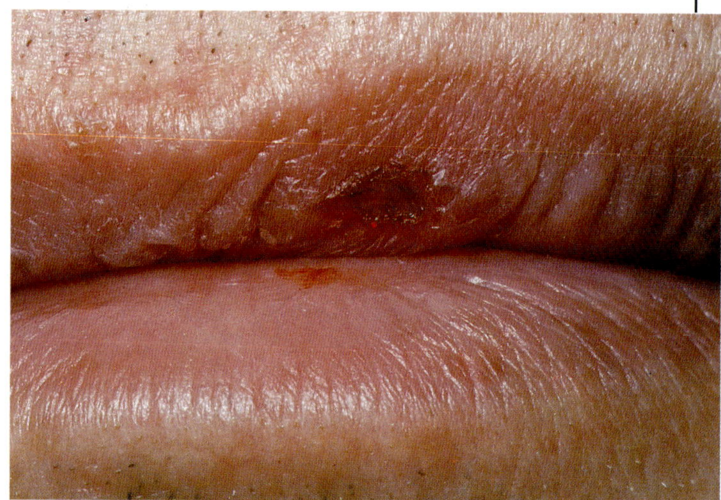

Vermillion Border

- Burn injury secondary to:
  - —inadequate bur protection
  - —heated instrument
  - —stretching and manipulation
  - —inadequate lubrication

Trauma to the Flap

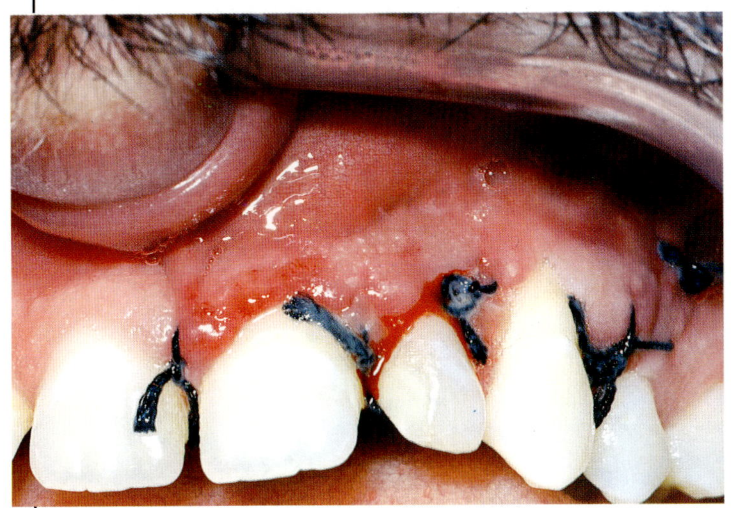

- Torn sutures:
  - — suture placement impinging on free gingival margin
  - — sutures placed under tension
  - — toothbrush trauma

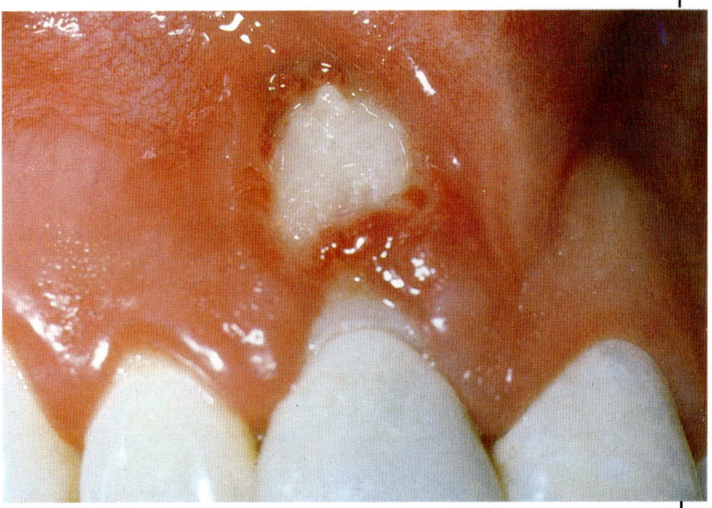

- Incision placed over root eminence.
- Suture placed under tension.

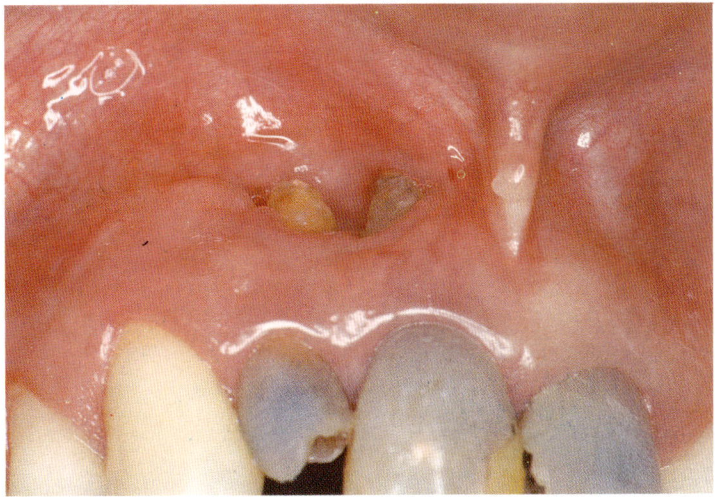

- Semilunar incision made over bony defect.
- Protruding root eminence in area of defect.

Malpositioned Retrograde Obturation Material

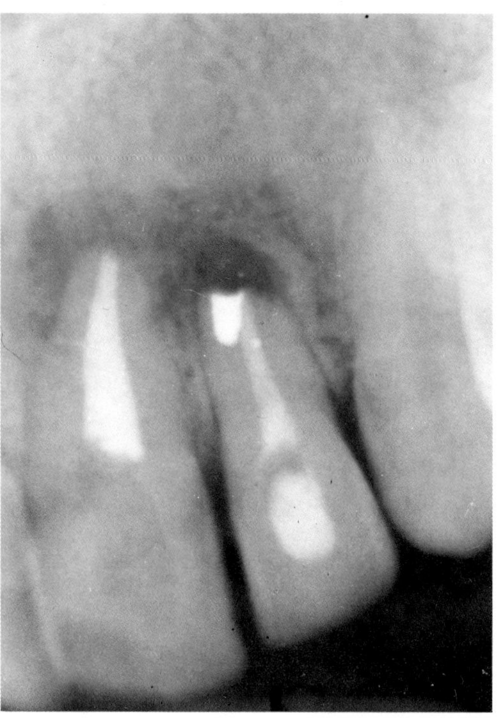

- Not in line with long axis of the root.
- Near perforation during apical preparation.

Incomplete Root Resection

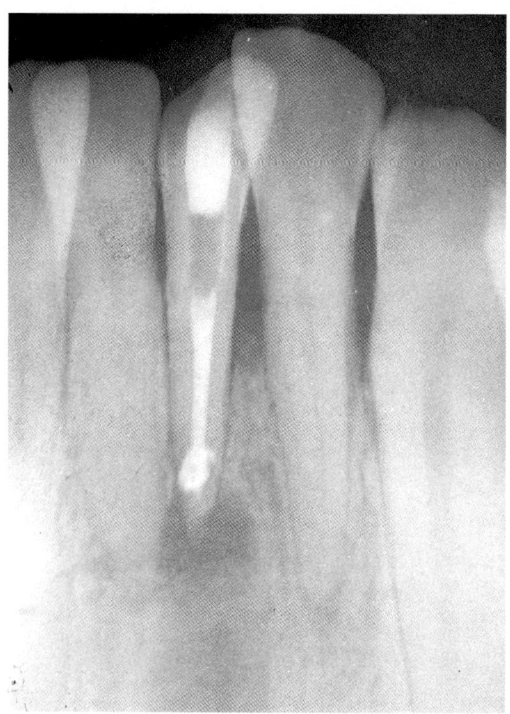

- Partial resection:
  - inadequate access
  - failure to define root before resection
  - closure made before radiographic confirmation

Foreign Debris in Surgical Site

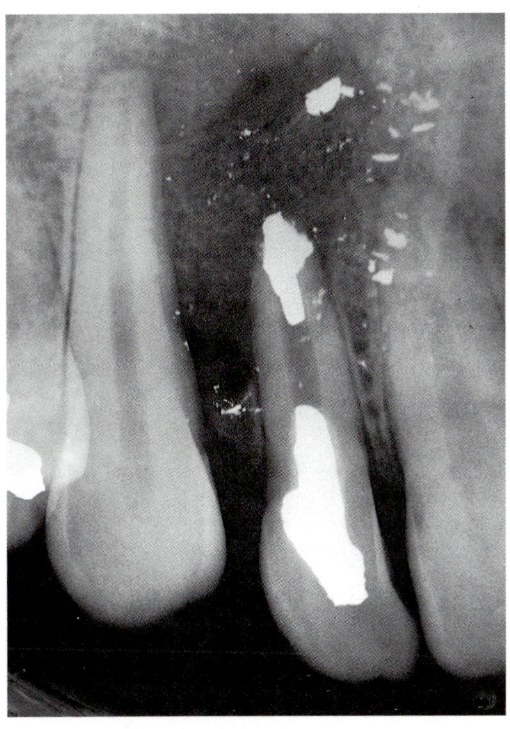

- Amalgam splatter:
  - improper handling of retrograde material
  - inadequate isolation and debridement
  - closure made before radiographic confirmation

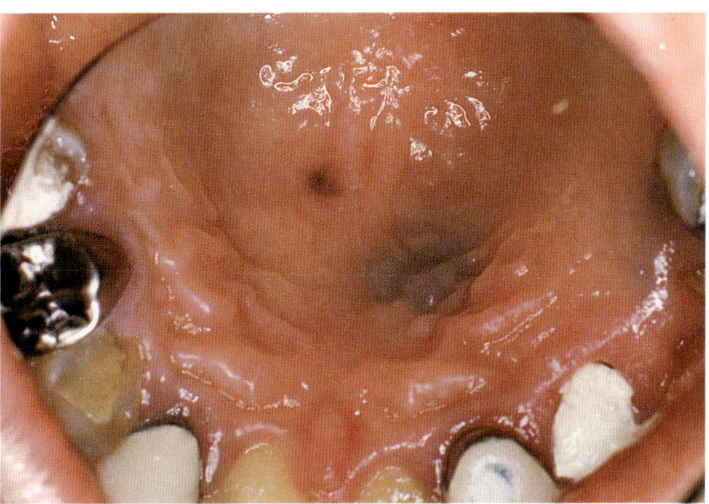

- Amalgam tattoo: amalgam particles remain in surgical site.

Paresthesia of the Lip

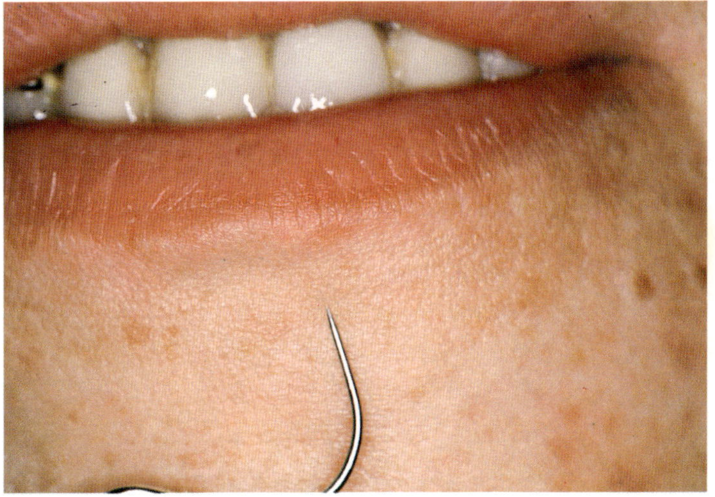

- Evaluate clinical extent.
- Surgical trauma:
  - impingement on mental nerve during reflection
  - incision trauma
  - pressure secondary to postsurgical swelling
  - trauma to mandibular nerve

Suggested Readings

Presurgical preparation

Bhaskar S. *Synopsis of Oral Pathology.* 7th ed. St Louis: CV Mosby Co; 1986.

Block S. *Disinfection, Sterilization and Preservation.* 3rd ed. Philadelphia: Lea & Febiger; 1983.

Eversole LR. *Clinical Outline of Oral Pathology: Diagnosis and Treatment.* 2nd ed. Philadelphia: Lea & Febiger; 1984: 203-250.

Holroyd SV, Wynn RL. *Clinical Pharmacology in Dental Practice.* 4th ed. St Louis: CV Mosby Co; 1988.

Little JW, Falace DA. *Dental Management of the Medically Compromised Patient.* 3rd ed. St Louis: CV Mosby Co; 1988.

Malamed S. *Handbook of Local Anesthesia.* 2nd ed. St Louis: CV Mosby Co; 1986.

Malamed S. *Handbook of Medical Emergencies in the Dental Office.* 3rd ed. St Louis: CV Mosby Co; 1987.

Maseman DC, Whetstone SD. Medical history review prior to local anesthesia administration. *Dental Hygiene* 1988; March: 131-135.

Physicians' Desk Reference. 44th ed. Oradell, NJ: Medical Economics Company Inc; 1990.

Robertson PB, Greenspan JS (eds). *Oral Manifestations of AIDS.* Littleton, Mass: PSG Publishing Company, Inc; 1988.

Flap design and suturing

Clarke MA, Bueltman KW. Anatomical considerations in periodontal surgery. *J Periodontol* 1971; 42: 610-625.

Dahlberg WH. Incisions and suturing: Some basic considerations about each in periodontal flap surgery. *Dent Clin North Am* 1969; 13: 149-159.

Davis JW, et al. Periodontal surgery as an adjunct to endodontics, orthodontics and restorative dentistry. *J Am Dent Assoc* 1987; 115: 271-275.

Holmes CH, Strem BE. Location of flap margin after suturing. *J Periodontol* 1976; 47: 674-675.

Kramper BJ, et al. A comparative study of the wound healing of three types of flap design used in periapical surgery. *J Endodont* 1984; 10: 17-25.

Lang NP, Löe H. The relationship between the width of keratinized gingiva and gingival health. *J Periodontol* 1972; 42: 423-427.

Lilly GE, et al. Reaction of oral tissues to suture materials, Parts II, III, IV. *Oral Surg* 1968; 26:592-599/ 1969; 28: 432-438/1972; 33: 152-157.

Macht SD, Krizek TJ. Sutures and suturing—Current concepts. *J Oral Surg* 1978; 36: 710.

Myer RD, Antonini CJ. A review of suture materials, Part I. *Compend Contin Educ Dent* 1989; (9)5: 260-264.

Myer RD, Antonini CJ. A review of suture materials, Part II. *Compend Contin Educ Dent* 1989; (9)6: 360-366.

Rakusin J, Harisson J. Alteration of the manipulative properties of plain gut suture material by hydration. *J Endodont* 1988; 4: 121-124.

Thacker JG, et al. Mechanical performance of surgical sutures. *Am J Surg* 1975; 130: 374.

Trephination/incision and drainage

Laskin DM. Anatomic considerations in diagnosis and treatment of odontogenic infections. *J Am Dent Assoc* 1964; 69: 308-316.

Peters DD. Evaluation of prophylactic alveolar trephination to avoid pain. *J Endodont* 1980; 6: 518-526.

Spilka CJ. Pathways of dental infections. *J Oral Surg* 1966; 24: 111-124.

Topazian RG, Goldberg MH. *Oral and Maxillofacial Infections.* 2nd ed. Philadelphia: WB Saunders Co; 1987.

Decompression

Freedland JB. Conservative reduction of large periapical lesions. *Oral Surg* 1970; 29: 455-464.

Kehoe JC. Decompression of a large periapical lesion: A short treatment course. *J Endodont* 1986; 12: 311-314.

Neaverth EJ, Burg HA. Decompression of large periapical cystic lesions. *J Endodont* 1982; 8: 175-182.

Patterson SS. Endodontic therapy: Use of a polyethylene tube and stint for drainage. *J Am Dent Assoc* 1964; 69: 710-714.

Samuels HS. Marsupialization: Effective management

of large maxillary cysts. *Oral Surg* 1965; 20: 676-683.

Walker TL, Davis MS. Treatment of large periapical lesions using cannulization through the involved teeth. *J Endodont* 1984; 10: 215-220.

Surgical endodontic techniques

Arens DE, Adams WR, De Castro, RA. *Endodontic Surgery.* Philadelphia: Harper and Row; 1981.

Bellizzi R. A teaching aid for maxillary molar palatal root surgery using an in vitro model. *J Endodont* 1983; 9: 398-401.

Block RM, Bushell A. Retrograde amalgam procedures for mandibular posterior teeth. *J Endodont* 1982; 8: 107-112.

Block RM, Lewis RD. Surgical treatment of iatrogenic canal blockages. *Oral Surg* 1987; 63: 722-732.

Cohn SA. The advantages of the greater palatine foramen block technique. *J Endodont* 1986; 12: 268-269.

Ericson S, et al. Results of apicoectomy of maxillary canines, premolars and molars with special reference to oral antral communications as a prognostic factor. *Int J Oral Surg* 1974; 3: 386-393.

Fishel D, et al. Roentgenologic study of the mental foramen. *Oral Surg* 1976; 41: 682-686.

Frank VH. Mandibular canal localization. *Oral Surg* 1966; 21: 312-315.

Gutmann JL. Principles of endodontic surgery for the general practitioner. *Dent Clin North Am* 1984; 28: 895-908.

Gutmann JL, Harrison JW. Posterior endodontic surgery: Anatomical considerations and clinical techniques. *Int Endod J* 1985; 18: 8-34.

Ibarrola JL, et al. Osseous reactions to three hemostatic agents. *J Endodont* 1985; 11: 75-83.

Ioannides C, Borstlap WA. Apicoectomy on molars: A clinical and radiographical study. *Int J Oral Surg* 1983; 12: 73-79.

Kruger GO. *Text Book of Oral and Maxillofacial Surgery.* 5th ed. St Louis: CV Mosby Co; 1979.

Lin L, et al. Oroantral communication in periapical surgery of maxillary posterior teeth. *J Endodont* 1985; 11: 40-44.

Littner MM, et al. Relationship between the apices of the lower molars and mandibular canal—A radiographic study. *Oral Surg* 1989; 62: 595-602.

Persson G. Periapical surgery of molars. *Int J Oral Surg* 1982; 11: 96-100.

Phillips JL, Weller RN, Kulild JC. The mental foramen: Part I. Size, orientation, and positional relationship to the mandibular second premolar. *J Endodont* 1990; 16: 221-223.

Rud J, et al. A follow-up study of 1000 cases treated by endodontic surgery. *Int J Oral Surg* 1972; 1: 215-228.

Selden HS. Bone wax as an effective hemostat in periapical surgery. *Oral Surg* 1970; 29: 262-264.

Selden HS. The endo-antral syndrome: An endodontic complication. *J Am Dent Assoc* 1989; 119: 397-402.

Selden HS, August D. Maxillary sinus involvement and endodontic complications. *Oral Surg* 1970; 30: 117.

Sweet APS. Radiodontic study of the mental foramen. *Dent Radiol Photo* 1959; 32: 28, 32-33.

Tebo HG, Telford IR. An analysis of the variations in position of the mental foramen. *Dent Items* 1951; 73: 52-53.

Retrograde obturation materials

Bondra DL, et al. Leakage in vitro with IRM, high copper amalgam and EBA cement as retrofilling materials. *J Endodont* 1989; 15: 157-160.

MacPherson MG, et al. Leakage in vitro with high-temperature thermoplasticized gutta-percha, high copper amalgam, and warm gutta-percha when used as retrofilling materials. *J Endodont* 1989; 15: 212-215.

Smee G, et al. Comparative leakage study of P-30 resin bonded ceramic, teflon, amalgam, and IRM as retrofilling seals. *J Endodont* 1987; 13: 117-121.

Szeremeta-Brown TL, et al. A comparison of the sealing properties of different retrograde techniques: An autoradiographic study. *Oral Surg* 1985; 59: 82-87.

Tronstad L, et al. Sealing ability of dental amalgams as retrograde fillings in endodontic therapy. *J Endodont* 1983; 9: 551-553.

Postsurgical complications

Buckley MJ, et al. Orbital emphysema causing vision loss after a dental extraction. *J Am Dent Assoc* 1990; 120: 421-424.

Donoghue R, et al. Etidocaine hydrochloride in surgical procedures: Effects on postoperative analgesia. *J Am Dent Assoc* 1990; 120: 429-434.

Reznick JB, Ardary WC. Cervicofacial subcutaneous air emphysema after dental extraction. *J Am Dent Assoc* 1990; 120: 417-419.

Appendix

Selected Manufacturers Listing

Advanced Dental Concepts, Inc
1 South Pickney Street
Madison, WI 53703
- Visual magnification

Almore Binocular Loupe
PO Box 25214
Portland, OR 97225
- Visual magnification

R. Beaver, Inc
PO Box 9097
411 Waverly Oaks Road
Waltham, MA 02254
- Beaver surgical blade handles
- Beaver surgical blades

Becton-Dickinson
PO Box 845
Rutherford, NJ 07070
- Luer-Lok syringe

L. D. Caulk Co
PO Box 359
Milford, DE 19963-0359
- IRM

Davol, Inc
Subsidiary of C.R. Bard, Inc
100 Sockanossett Crossroad
Cranston, RI 02920
- Penrose drains

Donegan Optical Company, Inc
15549 West 108th Street
Lenexa, KS 66219
- Visual magnification

Ethicon
PO Box 151
Somerville, NJ 08876-0151
- Bone wax
- 4-0 gut suture
- 4-0 silk suture

Halbran, Inc
PO Box 272
Willoughby, OH 44094
- Toothette disposable toothbrush

Hall Surgical
1170 Mark Avenue
Carpinteria, CA 46580
- Surgical drill

Hu-Friedy
3232 N Rockwell Street
Chicago, IL 60618
- no. 4 Molt curet
- no. 2 Molt curet

Johnson & Johnson Dental Care Company
ESDP Distribution Center
Room EE, 291A
Route 1
New Brunswick, NJ 08902
- Nu Gauze
- Surgicel

Marion Scientific
A Division of Marion Laboratories, Inc
Kansas City, MO 64114
- Anaerobic culturette

Procter & Gamble
PO Box 171
Cincinnati, OH 45202
- Peridex

Quality Aspirators
PO Box 382120
Duncanville, TX 75138-2120
- Fiberoptics

Union Broach
1107 Broadway
New York, NY 10010
- Apical file holder
- Microhead handpiece
- KG retrofilling amalgam carrier

UpJohn Company
700 Portage Road
Kalamazoo, MI 49001
- Gelfoam

Index